Lecture Notes in Computer Science 13746

More information about this series at https://link.springer.com/bookseries/558

Yufei Chen · Marius George Linguraru ·
Raj Shekhar · Stefan Wesarg · Marius Erdt ·
Klaus Drechsler · Cristina Oyarzun Laura (Eds.)

Clinical Image-Based Procedures

11th Workshop, CLIP 2022
Held in Conjunction with MICCAI 2022
Singapore, September 18, 2022
Proceedings

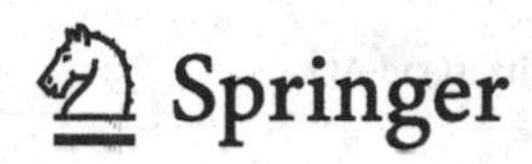

Editors
Yufei Chen
Tongji University
Shanghai, China

Raj Shekhar
Children's National Health System
Washington, DC, USA

Marius Erdt
Fraunhofer Singapore
Singapore, Singapore

Cristina Oyarzun Laura
Fraunhofer IGD
Darmstadt, Germany

Marius George Linguraru
Children's National Health System
Washington, DC, USA

Stefan Wesarg
Fraunhofer IGD
Darmstadt, Germany

Klaus Drechsler
Aachen University of Applied Sciences
Aachen, Germany

ISSN 0302-9743 ISSN 1611-3349 (electronic)
Lecture Notes in Computer Science
ISBN 978-3-031-23178-0 ISBN 978-3-031-23179-7 (eBook)
https://doi.org/10.1007/978-3-031-23179-7

This Springer imprint is published by the registered company Springer Nature Switzerland AG
The registered company address is: Gewerbestrasse 11, 6330 Cham, Switzerland

Preface

The 11th International Workshop on Clinical Image-based Procedures: Towards Holistic Patient Models for Personalised Healthcare (CLIP) was held on September 18, 2022, in conjunction with the 25th International Conference on Medical Image Computing and Computer Assisted Intervention (MICCAI 2022).

Following the long tradition of CLIP on translational research, the goal of the works presented in this workshop is to bring basic research methods closer to the clinical practice. One of the key aspects that is gaining relevance regarding the applicability of basic research methods in clinical practice is the creation of Holistic Patient Models as an important step towards personalised healthcare. As a matter of fact, the clinical picture of a patient does not uniquely consist of medical images, but a combination of medical image data of multiple modalities with other patient data, e.g., omics, demographics or electronic health records is desirable. Since 2019 CLIP has put a special emphasis on this area of research.

CLIP 2022 received 12 submissions and 9 of them were accepted for publication. All submitted papers were peer-reviewed by at least 3 experts. All accepted papers were presented by their authors during the workshop and the attendees chose with their votes the holder of the Best Paper Award of CLIP 2022. In addition to the oral presentations provided by the authors of the accepted papers, all attendees of CLIP 2022 had the opportunity to enjoy high-quality keynotes followed by avid discussions in which all attendees were involved. We would like to thank our invited speakers for their interesting talks and discussions:

Prof. Xiahai Zhuang, Fudan University, Shanghai, China, "Using Statistical Learning to Improve Interpretation and Generalization in Medical Image Computing and Analysis" (online).

Dr. Moti Freiman, Technion, Israel, "MR Physics Driven Artificial Intelligence" (on-site).

Furthermore, we would like to take this opportunity to thank also our program committee members, authors and attendees who helped CLIP 2022 to be a great success.

September 2022

Yufei Chen
Marius George Linguraru
Raj Shekhar
Stefan Wesarg
Marius Erdt
Klaus Drechsler
Cristina Oyarzun Laura

Organization

Organizing Committee

Yufei Chen	Tongji University, Shanghai, China
Klaus Drechsler	Aachen University of Applied Sciences, Germany
Marius Erdt	Fraunhofer Singapore, Singapore
Marius George Linguraru	Children's National Healthcare System, USA
Cristina Oyarzun Laura	Fraunhofer IGD, Germany
Raj Shekhar	Children's National Healthcare System, USA
Stefan Wesarg	Fraunhofer IGD, Germany

Program Committee

Niklas Babendererde	Technical University Darmstadt, Germany
Jan Egger	Graz University of Technology, Austria
Moti Freiman	Technion - Israel Institute of Technology, Israel
Moritz Fuchs	Technical University Darmstadt, Germany
Camila Gonzalez	Technical University Darmstadt, Germany
Anna-Sophia Hertlein	Fraunhofer IGD, Germany
Katarzyna Heryan	University of Science and Technology, Poland
Martin Hoßbach	Clear Guide Medical, USA
Yogesh Karpate	Chistats Labs Private Limited, India
Purnima Rajan	Clear Guide Medical, USA
Andreas Wirtz	Fraunhofer IGD, Germany
Lukas Zerweck	Fraunhofer ITMP, Germany
Stephan Zidowitz	Fraunhofer MEVIS, Germany

Contents

Fast Auto-differentiable Digitally Reconstructed Radiographs for Solving Inverse Problems in Intraoperative Imaging

Vivek Gopalakrishnan[1,2](✉) and Polina Golland[1,2]

[1] Harvard-MIT Health Sciences and Technology, Massachusetts Institute of Technology, Cambridge, MA, USA
[2] Computer Science and Artificial Intelligence Laboratory, Massachusetts Institute of Technology, Cambridge, MA, USA
{vivekg,polina}@csail.mit.edu

Abstract. The use of digitally reconstructed radiographs (DRRs) to solve inverse problems such as slice-to-volume registration and 3D reconstruction is well-studied in preoperative settings. In intraoperative imaging, the utility of DRRs is limited by the challenges in generating them in real-time and supporting optimization procedures that rely on repeated DRR synthesis. While immense progress has been made in accelerating the generation of DRRs through algorithmic refinements and GPU implementations, DRR-based optimization remains slow because most DRR generators do not offer a straightforward way to obtain gradients with respect to the imaging parameters. To make DRRs interoperable with gradient-based optimization and deep learning frameworks, we have reformulated Siddon's method, the most popular ray-tracing algorithm used in DRR generation, as a series of vectorized tensor operations. We implemented this vectorized version of Siddon's method in PyTorch, taking advantage of the library's strong automatic differentiation engine to make this DRR generator fully differentiable with respect to its parameters. Additionally, using GPU-accelerated tensor computation enables our vectorized implementation to achieve rendering speeds equivalent to state-of-the-art DRR generators implemented in CUDA and C++. We illustrate the resulting method in the context of slice-to-volume registration. Moreover, our simulations suggest that the loss landscapes for the slice-to-volume registration problem are convex in the neighborhood of the optimal solution, and gradient-based registration promises a much faster solution than prevailing gradient-free optimization strategies. The proposed DRR generator enables fast computer vision algorithms to support image guidance in minimally invasive procedures. Our implementation is publically available at https://github.com/v715/DiffDRR.

Keywords: DRRs · Differentiable programming · Inverse problems

Y. Chen et al. (Eds.): CLIP 2022, LNCS 13746, pp. 1–11, 2023.
https://doi.org/10.1007/978-3-031-23179-7_1

1 Introduction

Digitally reconstructed radiographs (DRRs) are simulated 2D X-ray images generated from 3D computational tomography (CT) volumes using a variety of ray-tracing techniques. While DRRs are widely used in preoperative settings (e.g., optimizing dose delivery in radiation oncology), many potentially valuable intraoperative use cases (e.g., real-time multimodal registration for image-guided procedures) are infeasible due to computational bottlenecks in generating DRRs and using them in slice-to-volume registration. Most open-source CPU-based implementations take about 1 s to generate a single DRR [9], which is not fast enough for intraoperative imaging systems with sampling rates of about 7.5 frames per second [8]. Numerous GPU-accelerated DRR generators have been proposed with run times on the order of 100 ms [1,5,7], but to the best of our knowledge, no publically available implementation exists.

The second limitation of currently available DRR generators is that it is challenging to efficiently compute derivatives using these renderers because they are implemented in low-level languages such as CUDA and C++. DRR generators are often used in conjunction with numerical optimization schemes to solve fundamental medical imaging problems (e.g., slice-to-volume registration), and the difficulty in computing derivatives means that gradient-based optimization techniques are often infeasible [13]. While many end-to-end deep learning approaches can solve X-ray to CT registration problems with high accuracy [2,3], these methods often require large amounts of training data, which can make them impractical for specialized interventional problems. Instead, many applications use iterative gradient-free methods, such as the Nelder-Mead method [11], to optimize an image similarity metric with respect to the parameters of the DRR generator [3,13]. While these methods are effective for optimizing highly nonlinear loss functions, we show that the loss landscapes for slice-to-volume registration in particular is convex in a large region around the optimum, making this problem better suited for gradient-based optimization methods.

We present a fast vectorized renderer that generates DRRs and their derivatives with respect to image geometry parameters automatically. We utilize PyTorch as a GPU-accelerated tensor algebra library with robust source-to-source automatic differentiation to implement differentiable DRRs. That is, using our implementation, DRR generation can be used as a differential operator to train deep learning algorithms for fast reconstruction and registration algorithms. We analyze the performance of our implementation and the correctness of the automatically obtained derivatives, and demonstrate an experiment where our differentiable DRR generator solves a slice-to-volume registration problem. Our hope is that this open-source package will be useful for translating computer vision algorithms to real-time implementations for interventional applications.

2 Methods

We start by summarizing Siddon's method [10], commonly used for ray-tracing in DRR synthesis, and its extensions that accelerate rendering speed. We then

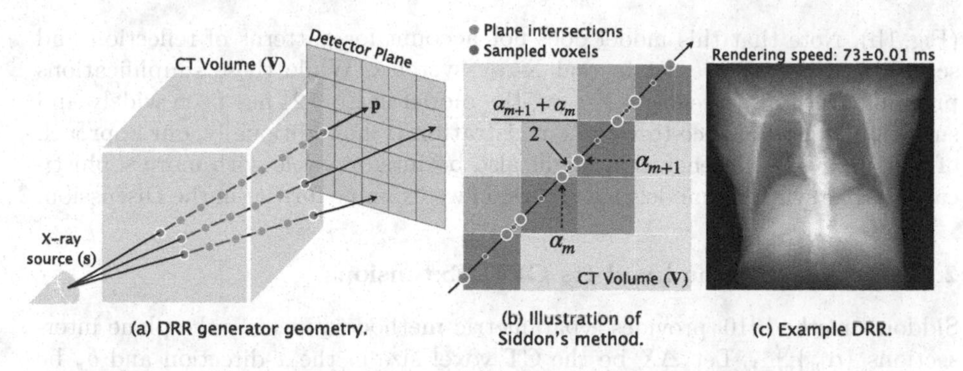

Fig. 1. DRR synthesis. (a) We assume an idealized model of a projectional radiography imaging system: X-ray beams are emitted with a fixed initial energy from a point source $\mathbf{s} \in \mathbb{R}^3$, beam energy diminishes as the X-rays travel through the CT volume $\mathbf{V}$, and energy in the attenuated beams is measured when the X-rays hit a point on the detector $\mathbf{p} \in \mathbb{R}^3$, producing the DRR. (b) In Siddon's method, the image location value at $\mathbf{p}$ is a weighted average of the intensities of the voxels through which the ray passes, where the weight is the length of the ray's intersection with the voxel. The values α_m and α_{m+1} parameterize the intersection of the ray with two adjacent planes, and the midpoint $\frac{\alpha_{m+1}+\alpha_m}{2}$ identifies the current voxel through which the ray is passing. (c) Our vectorized Siddon's method generates a 200×200 DRR in $72.7\,\mathrm{ms} \pm 10\,\mu\mathrm{s}$ on an NVIDIA GeForce RTX 2080 Ti.

describe our vectorized implementation of Siddon's method, which achieves rendering speeds equivalent to those of existing GPU-accelerated methods while also being fully differentiable.

2.1 DRR Generation

The process of generating a DRR models the geometry of an idealized projectional radiography system (Fig. 1a). Let $\mathbf{s} \in \mathbb{R}^3$ be the X-ray source, and $\mathbf{p} \in \mathbb{R}^3$ be a target pixel on the detector plane. Then $R(\alpha) = \mathbf{s} + \alpha(\mathbf{p} - \mathbf{s})$ is a ray that originates from $\mathbf{s}$ ($\alpha = 0$), passes through the imaged volume, and hits the detector plane at $\mathbf{p}$ ($\alpha = 1$). The total energy attenuation experienced by the X-ray by the time it reaches pixel $\mathbf{p}$ is given by the following line integral:

$$E(R) = \|\mathbf{p} - \mathbf{s}\|_2 \int_0^1 \mathbf{V}(\mathbf{s} + \alpha(\mathbf{p} - \mathbf{s}))\, \mathrm{d}\alpha, \tag{1}$$

where $\mathbf{V} : \mathbb{R}^3 \mapsto \mathbb{R}$ is the imaged volume. The term $\|\mathbf{p}-\mathbf{s}\|_2$ endows the unit-free $\mathrm{d}\alpha$ with the physical unit of length. For DRR synthesis, $\mathbf{V}$ is approximated by a discrete 3D CT volume, and Eq. (1) becomes

$$E(R) = \|\mathbf{p} - \mathbf{s}\|_2 \sum_{m=1}^{M-1} (\alpha_{m+1} - \alpha_m) \mathbf{V}\left[\mathbf{s} + \frac{\alpha_{m+1} + \alpha_m}{2}(\mathbf{p} - \mathbf{s})\right], \tag{2}$$

where α_m parameterizes the locations where ray R intersects one of the orthogonal planes comprising the CT volume, and M is the number of such intersections

(Fig. 1b). Note that this model does not account for patterns of reflection and scattering that are present in real X-ray systems. While these simplifications preclude synthesis of realistic X-rays, the model in Eq. (2) has been widely and successfully used in slice-to-volume registration [13]. Additionally, our approach of vectorizing DRR generation might also be interoperable with more sophisticated image synthesis models, an extension we examine further in the Discussion.

2.2 Siddon's Method and Its GPU Extensions

Siddon's method [10] provides a parametric method to identify the plane intersections $\{\alpha_m\}_{m=1}^M$. Let ΔX be the CT voxel size in the x-direction and b_x be the location of the 0-th plane in this direction. Then the intersection of ray R with the i-th plane in the x-direction is given by

$$\alpha_x(i) = \frac{b_x + i\Delta X - \mathbf{s}_x}{\mathbf{p}_x - \mathbf{s}_x}, \tag{3}$$

with analogous expressions for $\alpha_y(\cdot)$ and $\alpha_z(\cdot)$. We can use Eq. (3) to compute the values $\boldsymbol{\alpha}_x$ for all the intersections between R and the planes in the x-direction:

$$\boldsymbol{\alpha}_x = \{\alpha_x(i_{\min}), \dots, \alpha_x(i_{\max})\},$$

where $i_{\min}$ and $i_{\max}$ denote the first and last intersections of R with the x-direction planes. Defining $\boldsymbol{\alpha}_y$ and $\boldsymbol{\alpha}_z$ analogously, we construct the array

$$\boldsymbol{\alpha} = \mathrm{sort}(\boldsymbol{\alpha}_x, \boldsymbol{\alpha}_y, \boldsymbol{\alpha}_z), \tag{4}$$

which contains M values of α parameterizing the intersections between R and the orthogonal x-, y-, and z-directional planes. We substitute values in the sorted set $\boldsymbol{\alpha}$ into Eq. (2) to evaluate $E(R)$, which corresponds to the intensity of pixel $\mathbf{p}$ in the synthesized DRR.

A faster variant determines consecutive intersecting planes iteratively [4]. For example, the value of α at the second plane intersected by R is given by $\alpha_2 = \min\{\alpha_x(i_{\min}+1), \alpha_y(j_{\min}+1), \alpha_z(k_{\min}+1)\}$. The algorithm iteratively finds the next value of α until we reach the edge of the CT volume, making this approach more memory efficient by requiring fewer intermediate values to be stored. This modified algorithm, known as Siddon-Jacobs' method, is commonly implemented in CUDA and C++ to create multi-threaded GPU-accelerated DRR generators that exploit data parallelism by assigning each thread to trace an independent ray intersecting the detector plane [1,5,7].

2.3 Vectorizing Siddon's Method

While Siddon-Jacobs' method is more memory efficient, the iterative loop it relies on is not amenable to implementations in vectorized tensor algebra libraries. Thus we vectorize the original Siddon's method as follows. Let $\mathbf{P} \in \mathbb{R}^{H \times W \times 3}$ contain the 3D pixel coordinates of a DRR with dimension $H \times W$. We compute the α values for intersections with all of the x-, y-, and z-planes for all $\mathbf{p} \in \mathbf{P}$ in parallel:

$$\mathbf{A} = \left(\left(\begin{pmatrix} b_x \\ b_y \\ b_z \end{pmatrix} + \begin{pmatrix} i \\ j \\ k \end{pmatrix} \otimes \begin{pmatrix} \Delta X \\ \Delta Y \\ \Delta Z \end{pmatrix} \right) - \mathbf{s} \right) \oslash (\mathbf{P} - \mathbf{s}) \in \mathbb{R}^{H \times W \times (n_x + n_y + n_z)}, \quad (5)$$

where (n_x, n_y, n_z) are the dimensions of the CT volume $\mathbf{V}$, (i, j, k) are the CT voxel indices, $(\Delta X, \Delta Y, \Delta Z)$ are the CT voxel sizes, and $\otimes$ and $\oslash$ are the Hadamard product and division operators, respectively. Rather than explicitly compute the indices $(i_{\min}, i_{\max})$, $(j_{\min}, j_{\max})$, and $(k_{\min}, k_{\max})$ for each ray, as is done in Siddon's original method, we instead compute the minimum and maximum values of $\boldsymbol{\alpha}$, corresponding to when each ray enters and exits the volume:

$$\boldsymbol{\alpha}_{\min} = \max\left\{ \min\{\boldsymbol{\alpha}_x(0), \boldsymbol{\alpha}_x(n_x)\}, \min\{\boldsymbol{\alpha}_y(0), \boldsymbol{\alpha}_y(n_y)\}, \min\{\boldsymbol{\alpha}_z(0), \boldsymbol{\alpha}_z(n_z)\}\right\}$$
$$\boldsymbol{\alpha}_{\max} = \min\left\{ \max\{\boldsymbol{\alpha}_x(0), \boldsymbol{\alpha}_x(n_x)\}, \max\{\boldsymbol{\alpha}_y(0), \boldsymbol{\alpha}_y(n_y)\}, \max\{\boldsymbol{\alpha}_z(0), \boldsymbol{\alpha}_z(n_z)\}\right\},$$

where $\boldsymbol{\alpha}_{\min}, \boldsymbol{\alpha}_{\max} \in \mathbb{R}^{H \times W}$. We filter $\mathbf{A}$ to include only values in the range $[\boldsymbol{\alpha}_{\min}, \boldsymbol{\alpha}_{\max}]$ and sort each row $\mathbf{A}(h, w, \cdot)$ for $h \in \{1, \ldots, H\}, w \in \{1, \ldots, W\}$. Finally, we evaluate Eq. (2) with this sorted tensor to compute the intensity for each pixel in the DRR, completing a chain of vectorized tensor operations.

Because we reformulated the original Siddon's method as a series of tensor operations, our vectorized version benefits from the mature GPU compilers and memory allocators developed for optimizing large-scale deep learning models. For empirical evaluation of our method, we also implemented a partially-vectorized version of Siddon-Jacobs' method in which the α updates are still computed iteratively (i.e., with a loop), but the updates are applied in a vectorized form to every target pixel in the detector plane.

2.4 Differentiating DRRs with Respect to Imaging Parameters

We specify the 3D position of the X-ray source and detector plane relative to the CT volume with the following seven geometric parameters: radius ρ that acts as a scaling factor; three rotational degrees of freedom (DoF) $(\theta, \varphi, \gamma)$; and three translational DoF (b_x, b_y, b_z). Using spherical coordinates, we express the position of the X-ray source as $\mathbf{s} = (\rho, \theta, \varphi)$, where ρ is half of the source-to-detector distance, and θ and φ are the azimuthal and polar angles, respectively. We assume the detector plane is tangent to this implied sphere at the point opposite $\mathbf{s}$. The orientation of this plane is determined by a rotation about the x-axis by the angle γ. We add the translation (b_x, b_y, b_z) to the coordinates of the X-ray source and detector plane to create a reference frame wherein the patient is not perfectly centered relative to the X-ray scanner.

Since every step of our pipeline, from the generation of the pixels on the detector plane to the computation of the pixel intensities, is performed in PyTorch's tensor framework, the resulting DRRs are differentiable with respect to the parameters described above. That is, the gradient $\nabla_{\eta} \mathcal{L}(I(\boldsymbol{\eta}))$ of the loss function $\mathcal{L}(\cdot)$ evaluated for the DRR $I(\boldsymbol{\eta})$ with respect to the parameters $\boldsymbol{\eta} = (\rho, \theta, \varphi, \gamma, b_x, b_y, b_z)$ is obtained automatically for any differentiable $\mathcal{L}(\cdot)$.

3 Experiments

We evaluate the proposed efficient implementation of the algorithm on a reference chest CT scan from Slicer3D [6]. We compare the performance of the method to two baseline approaches and illustrate its application for gradient-based slice-to-volume registration.

3.1 Performance Analysis

We compare our vectorized GPU version of Siddon's method (VGS) to two baseline approaches: a widely used CPU implementation in the Plastimatch package (CP) [9], and our vectorized GPU implementation of Siddon-Jacobs' method (VGSJ) which we described in Sect. 2.3. Note that the CUDA-accelerated DRR generator in Plastimatch is not working at the time of publication. GPU benchmarks are run on an NVIDIA GeForce RTX 2080 Ti, and CPU benchmarks are run on an 18-core Linux computer with Intel(R) Xeon(R) CPU E5-2697 v4 @ 2.30 GHz processors.

Results. Table 1 summarizes statistics for the run time and accuracy of our method and the two baseline approaches, as well as intensity differences between our method and Plastimatch, and gradient differences between our method and FFD. Our implementation is much faster than Plastimatch, which is to be expected as Plastimatch is executed on the CPU. Numerically, the two implementations are very similar with an average root-mean-square error (RMSE) of $(8.3 \pm 1.9) \times 10^{-4}$ where the images are normalized to the range of $[0, 1]$. For DRRs smaller than $H = 500$, our method is faster than the vectorized version of Siddon-Jacobs' despite our method's high memory requirements. However, at $H = 500$, they have roughly equivalent run times. For smaller image sizes, our DRR generator achieves equivalent run times to previously reported GPU-accelerated implementations [1,5,7]. The gradients obtained via PyTorch auto-differentiation for our method are within 0.05 ± 0.01 of those computed via forward finite differences with a step size of 10^{-6} and are an order of magnitude more efficient to generate (35.1 ms ± 73.3 s *vs* 400.5 ms ± 821.4 s).

Table 1. Benchmark results. The dimension of the DRRs is $H \times W$. Each metric is averaged over 20 runs. (VGS = Vectorized GPU Siddon's method, VGSJ = Vectorized GPU Siddon-Jacobs' method, and CP = CPU Plastimatch.)

	Timing (ms)			RMSE	Autograd *vs* FFD
$H = W$	VGS	VGSJ	CP	VGS *vs* CP	VGS
100	**17.6 ± 0.05**	380 ± 20.9	1028 ± 132	$(6.9 \pm 2.2) \times 10^{-4}$	0.03 ± 0.02
200	**72.7 ± 0.01**	424 ± 4.2	1784 ± 488	$(8.7 \pm 2.7) \times 10^{-4}$	0.06 ± 0.01
300	**165 ± 0.13**	432 ± 19.2	2941 ± 821	$(6.4 \pm 1.2) \times 10^{-4}$	0.08 ± 0.02
400	**296 ± 0.06**	425 ± 2.8	6472 ± 643	$(9.0 \pm 1.9) \times 10^{-4}$	0.03 ± 0.005
500	453 ± 41.2	**425 ± 4.6**	8472 ± 478	$(11.7 \pm 4.3) \times 10^{-4}$	0.07 ± 0.006

3.2 DRR-Based Gradient Descent for Slice-to-Volume Registration

We use our auto-differentiable DRR generator to implement slice-to-volume registration with synthetic DRRs. Specifically, we generate a fixed DRR from a set of ground truth parameters $\boldsymbol{\eta}^* = (\theta, \varphi, \gamma, b_x, b_y, b_z)$, and generate a second moving DRR from a set of random initial parameters $\boldsymbol{\eta}_0$. We use basic gradient descent to minimize the negative Zero-Normalized Cross-Correlation (ZNCC) between the fixed DRR and the moving DRR.

Image Similarity Metrics are Locally Convex. First, we conduct a simulation study to show that the loss landscape generated by negative ZNCC is convex in a neighborhood around $\boldsymbol{\eta}^*$. We generate moving DRRs by sampling rotational and positional displacements. We sample all parameters uniformly from ranges of 90° for θ and φ, 45° for γ, and 30 mm for b_x, b_y, and b_z around the ground truth parameters $\boldsymbol{\eta}^*$. Although our generator provides gradients with respect to other model parameters like the source-to-detector distance (2ρ) and the DRR's dimensions and pixel spacing ($H, W, \Delta x, \Delta y$), we assume that those parameters are fixed (e.g., provided in the DICOM header), and instead focus our analysis on this 6 DoF registration problem. We observe that negative ZNCC is locally convex (Fig. 2), suggesting that it would be an apt loss function to optimize with gradient descent. We observed similar loss landscapes for the L^2 norm.

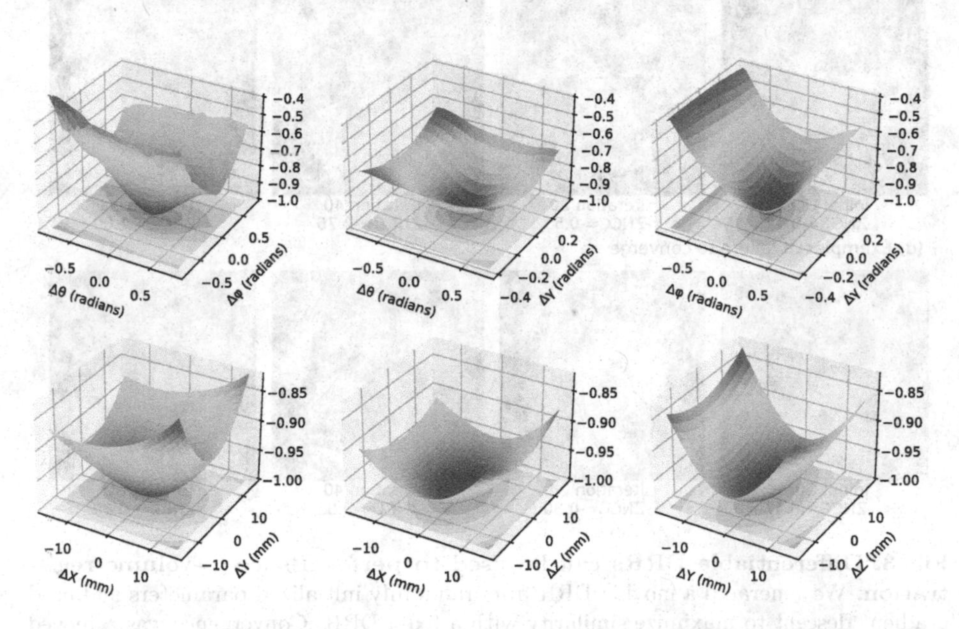

Fig. 2. Negative ZNCC is convex around the optimal DRR parameters. Rotational and positional displacements were sampled uniformly from ranges of 90° for θ and φ, 45° for γ, and 30 mm for b_x, b_y, and b_z.

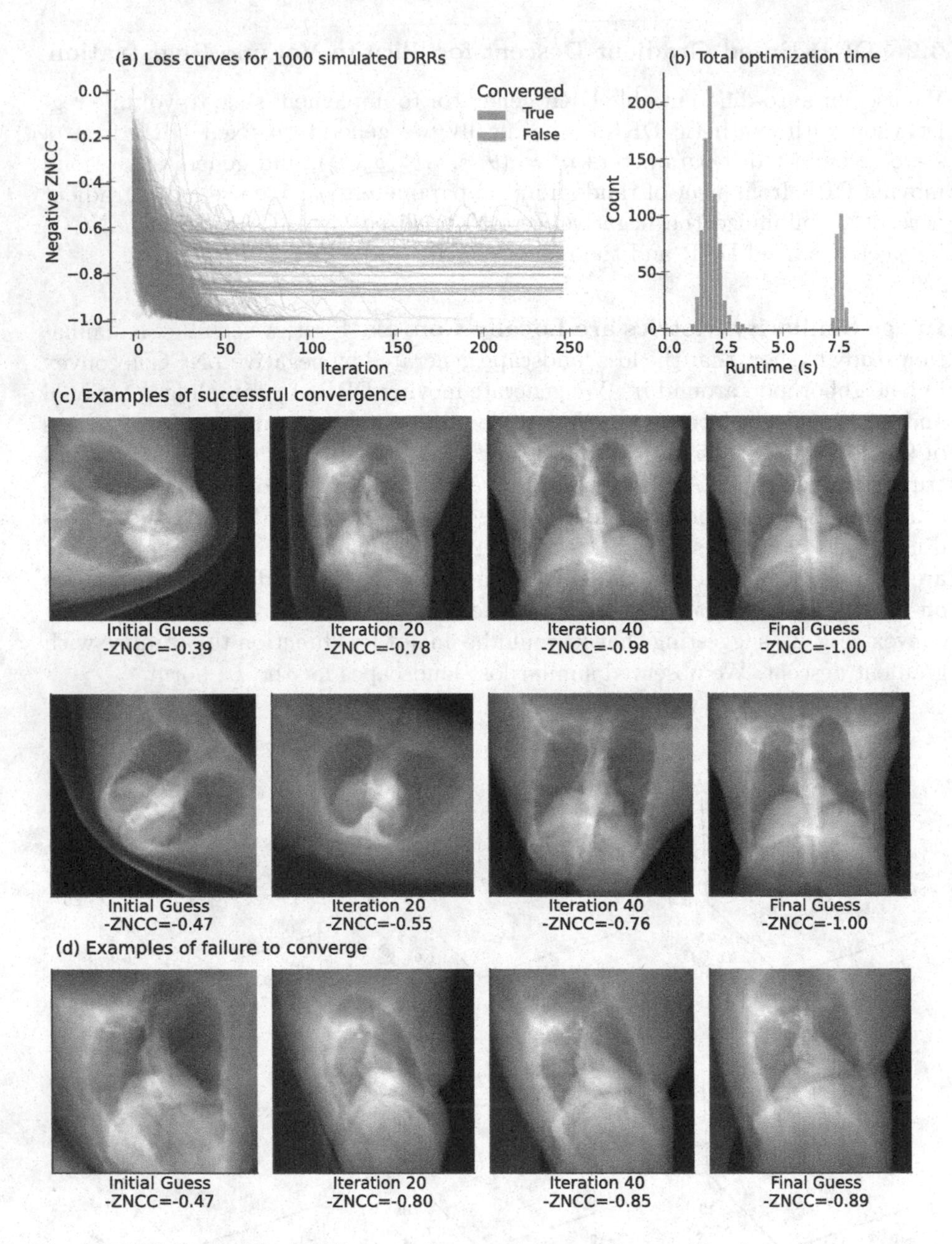

Fig. 3. Differentiable DRRs can be used to perform slice-to-volume registration. We generated a moving DRR from randomly initialized parameters and used gradient descent to maximize similarity with a fixed DRR. Convergence was achieved for 745/1000 simulated DRRs in an average 66 iterations (1.92 s). Examples of the optimization process are visualized at initial, intermediate (the 20th and 40th iterations), and final steps. DRRs for which convergence fails to occur get stuck in a local minimum with low negative ZNCC.

Differentiable DRR Registration Converges Quickly. Given a fixed DRR and a moving DRR, we optimized the parameters of the moving DRR with a basic implementation of gradient descent. We used different update rates for the rotational and translational parameters because they have different units ($\beta_{\theta\varphi\gamma} = 5.3 \times 10^{-2}$ and $\beta_{xyz} = 7.5 \times 10^{1}$), and momentum $\lambda = 0.9$. Additionally, to investigate the local minima in which our gradient descent algorithm could get stuck, we expanded the space of possible initializations beyond a convex neighborhood to 120° for θ, φ, and γ, and 60 mm for b_x, b_y, and b_z. The size of the CT volume is 360 mm × 360 mm × 332.5 mm.

For each randomly initialized DRR, we ran 250 iterations of gradient descent and determined that the moving DRR had converged to the fixed DRR if the negative ZNCC between the two images was less than −0.999. If this did not occur within 250 iterations, we treated the run as having failed to converge. Of the 1,000 randomly initialized DRRs we generated, 745 converged and 255 failed to converge (Fig. 3a). The initializations that converged solved the 6 DoF slice-to-volume registration problem 65.48 ± 14.27 iterations (1.92 ± 0.43 s).

We visualize multiple optimization steps for our gradient descent registration algorithm (Fig. 3c). From the examples that converged, our model successfully recovers the true pose parameters from challenging initializations, reaching a more reasonable estimate by the intermediate 20th iteration (Fig. 3b). In one example of an initialization that failed to converge, we see that the model gets stuck in a local minimum (Fig. 3c). In the final iteration in this example, the estimated DRR is orthogonal to the sagittal plane. The geometry of this scene looks similar to the coronal DRR (ground truth), giving the illusion of two lungs. We emphasize that our goal is not to propose a novel registration algorithm, but to provide an efficient DRR synthesis procedure that can support numerous downstream optimization applications, including registration.

4 Discussion

We present a fast auto-differentiable DRR generator that can be used to solve inverse problems in intraoperative imaging. By reformulating Siddon's method for ray-tracing through a CT volume as series of vectorized tensor operations, we obtain gradients of image loss functions with respect to DRR generating parameters while achieving rendering speeds equivalent to multi-threaded GPU-accelerated generators written in low-level languages such as CUDA and C++. This approach promises to enable fast solutions to DRR-based optimization problems with gradient methods, a strategy which was previously infeasible due to the inefficiency of generating gradients with finite differences. We demonstrate the effectiveness of this approach by solving a 6 DoF slice-to-volume registration problem using a locally convex image loss function.

Our future research on auto-differentiable DRRs will investigate their use in a deep learning framework to pre-train for specific intraoperative imaging tasks (e.g., spatiotemporal registration in interventional cardiology). Such pre-training could yield even faster solutions to inverse problems by finding better initializations or powering end-to-end models. One issue that might limit the effectiveness of such pre-training is that DRRs generated using Siddon's method are not realistic because they do not model any form of scattering. We will investigate fusing our method with DeepDRR [12], a deep learning framework that estimates scattering effects using Monte Carlo simulations, to produce DRRs that are simultaneously realistic, fast, and differentiable.

Acknowledgements. The authors thank Allie Forman for helpful feedback and support. This work was supported, in part, by NIH NIBIB 5T32EB1680, NIH NIBIB NAC P41EB015902, and NIH NINDS U19NS115388.

References

1. De Greef, M., Crezee, J., Van Eijk, J., Pool, R., Bel, A.: Accelerated ray tracing for radiotherapy dose calculations on a GPU. Med. Phys. **36**(9Part1), 4095–4102 (2009)
2. Esteban, J., Grimm, M., Unberath, M., Zahnd, G., Navab, N.: Towards fully automatic x-ray to ct registration. In: Shen, D., et al. (eds.) MICCAI 2019. LNCS, vol. 11769, pp. 631–639. Springer, Cham (2019). https://doi.org/10.1007/978-3-030-32226-7_70
3. Hou, B., et al.: Predicting slice-to-volume transformation in presence of arbitrary subject motion. In: Descoteaux, M., Maier-Hein, L., Franz, A., Jannin, P., Collins, D.L., Duchesne, S. (eds.) MICCAI 2017. LNCS, vol. 10434, pp. 296–304. Springer, Cham (2017). https://doi.org/10.1007/978-3-319-66185-8_34
4. Jacobs, F., Sundermann, E., De Sutter, B., Christiaens, M., Lemahieu, I.: A fast algorithm to calculate the exact radiological path through a pixel or voxel space. J. Comput. Inf. Technol. **6**(1), 89–94 (1998)
5. Mori, S., Kobayashi, M., Kumagai, M., Minohara, S.: Development of a GPU-based multithreaded software application to calculate digitally reconstructed radiographs for radiotherapy. Radiol. Phys. Technol. **2**(1), 40–45 (2008). https://doi.org/10.1007/s12194-008-0040-3
6. Pieper, S., Halle, M., Kikinis, R.: 3d slicer. In: 2004 2nd IEEE International Symposium on Biomedical Imaging: Nano to Macro, pp. 632–635. IEEE (2004)
7. Ruijters, D., ter Haar Romeny, B.M., Suetens, P.: GPU-accelerated digitally reconstructed radiographs. BioMED **8**, 431–435 (2008)
8. Sadamatsu, K., Nakano, Y.: The effect of low frame rate fluoroscopy on the x-ray dose during coronary intervention. Intern. Med. **55**(15), 1943–6 (2016)
9. Sharp, G.C., et al.: Plastimatch: an open source software suite for radiotherapy image processing. In: Proceedings of the XVI'th International Conference on the use of Computers in Radiotherapy (ICCR) (2010)
10. Siddon, R.L.: Fast calculation of the exact radiological path for a three-dimensional CT array. Med. Phys. **12**(2), 252–255 (1985)
11. Singer, S., Nelder, J.: Nelder-mead algorithm. Scholarpedia **4**(7), 2928 (2009)

12. Unberath, M., et al.: DeepDRR – a catalyst for machine learning in fluoroscopy-guided procedures. In: Frangi, A.F., Schnabel, J.A., Davatzikos, C., Alberola-López, C., Fichtinger, G. (eds.) MICCAI 2018. LNCS, vol. 11073, pp. 98–106. Springer, Cham (2018). https://doi.org/10.1007/978-3-030-00937-3_12
13. Van Der Bom, I., Klein, S., Staring, M., Homan, R., Bartels, L.W., Pluim, J.P.: Evaluation of optimization methods for intensity-based 2d–3d registration in x-ray guided interventions. In: Medical Imaging 2011: Image Processing, vol. 7962, pp. 657–671. SPIE (2011)

Multi-channel Residual Neural Network Based on Squeeze-and-Excitation for Osteoporosis Diagnosis

Chunmei Xia[1], Yue Ding[2,3], Jionglin Wu[2], Wenqiang Luo[2], Peidong Guo[2], Tianfu Wang[1], and Baiying Lei[1](✉)

[1] School of Biomedical Engineering, Health Science Center, National-Regional Key Technology Engineering Laboratory for Medical Ultrasound, Guangdong Key Laboratory for Biomedical Measurements and Ultrasound Imaging, Shenzhen University, Shenzhen 518060, China
leiby@szu.edu.cn

[2] Department of Orthopedics, Sun Yat-Sen Memorial Hospital, Sun Yat-Sen University, Guangzhou 510000, People's Republic of China

[3] Bioland Laboratory (Guangzhou Regenerative Medicine and Health Guangdong Laboratory), Guangzhou 510005, China

Abstract. Osteoporosis is a progressive, systemic skeletal disease, which is likely to occur in postmenopausal women. The osteoporosis detection utilizing bone mineral density (BMD) measurements by the dualenergy x-ray absorptiometry (DXA) device is expensive and highly ionizing. Bone quantitative ultrasound (QUS) has been regarded as a potential alternative for osteoporosis screening and diagnosis. However, the diagnosis accuracy of QUS is quite low using speed of sound (SOS). Currently, the deep learning method has shown powerful feature extraction capabilities from medical data. In order to improve the diagnosis accuracy of osteoporosis, we propose a multi-channel residual neural network via squeeze-and-excitation attention mechanism (MAResNet), which can extract discriminative features from radio-frequency (RF) signals generated from QUS. Compared with the conventional QUS method using SOS, experimental results indicate that our proposed method achieves superior performance, which can be beneficial to the osteoporosis screening.

Keywords: Multi-channel residual neural network · Osteoporosis diagnosis · Squeeze-and-excitation mechanism · Ultrasound radio frequency signals

1 Introduction

Osteoporosis is a systemic skeletal disease characterized by decreased bone mass and destruction of bone tissue microarchitecture, which increases the susceptibility to fracture [1]. Currently, the gold standard for osteoporosis detection

Y. Chen et al. (Eds.): CLIP 2022, LNCS 13746, pp. 12–21, 2023.
https://doi.org/10.1007/978-3-031-23179-7_2

utilizes bone mineral density (BMD) measurements, which is completed by the dualenergy x-ray absorptiometry (DXA) device, with the most frequently used measurement sites of the proximal femur, the lumbar spine, and the distal radius [2]. However, the measured value is sensitive to the posture of human body, and it fails to evaluate bone strength and microarchitecture [3]. Moreover, the DXA scanner has the disadvantages such as ionizing radiation, high inspection costs and inconvenience in movement. Consequently, DXA is currently difficult to popularize for osteoporosis screening and fracture risk assessment at primary health care [4].

Quantitative ultrasound (QUS) was first applied for osteoporosis and fracture assessment in 1984, with the advantages of low equipment cost, no radiation and portability [5]. QUS not only reflects bone density, but also correlates with mechanical properties of bone structure, bone elasticity and bone fragility. The speed of sound (SOS) is one of the common QUS parameters, which has a significant correlation with BMD [6]. Radius QUS measured by SOS is a potential alternative in geographies when DXA equipment is not available [7]. However, the accuracy of osteoporosis diagnosis using QUS is too low compared with DXA due to that QUS uses a simplified physical model of sound propagation in the bone for BMD measurement, which only extracts few features such as SOS from ultrasound signals [8,9].

The ultrasonic radio frequency (RF) signal generated from QUS device is an unfiltered native ultrasound signal, and the RF signal measured through the radius contains abundant tissue characteristics and structural information. However, the large amount of information in RF signals makes it difficult to analyze them using traditional algorithms. In order to explore the characteristics of RF signals, a more suitable model is required. Recently, the deep learning methods have shown powerful feature extraction abilities and can extract recognizable feature representations from data, which has been extensively studied in the field of one- dimensional data such as ECG, EEG and speech processing [10,11]. The deep learning method is first proposed in 2016, and the residual neural network (ResNet) is widely used due to its powerful ability to extract features from data, which mostly benefits from the residual connection [12,13]. Recently, the attention unit named squeeze-and-excitation (SE) was developed to emphasize the informative channel-wise feature [14]. Although deep learning methods have powerful analytical capabilities, as far as we know, few studies have been proposed for the diagnosis of osteoporosis based on deep learning and ultrasonic radiofrequency signals. Inspired by the advantage of ResNet and SE mechanism, we try to combine the SE module with ResNet to extract the most discriminative features of RF signals.

To address the above issues, we construct a multi-channel residual neural network via SE to explore the information of the RF signals of each channel. We first use MResnet to perform feature extraction for each channel, and then use the SE module to obtain more discriminative features by exploiting the correlation between channels. Overall, MAResNet based on ultrasound RF signals can capture the features of RF signals effectively for osteoporosis diagnosis. Our proposed method gets better osteoporosis diagnosis performance than conventional QUS method using SOS and some other deep learning methods, which is of great significance for osteoporosis screening.

2 Methodology

The QUS device used in this paper can receive 4 channels of data at the same time. For the RF source data collected by different channels, we design MResNet to analyze it. We combine multi-channel training with ResNet, and use SE unit to cascade the features extracted by the MResNet network in the channel direction. Specifically, the preliminary feature extraction is carried out by MResNet, and then the extracted features are fed into the SE unit for feature recalibration, which can better capture differences and correlations between different channels and remove redundant features. The recalibrated features are input into the fully connected layer for the osteoporosis classification. Meanwhile, we investigated the impact of the main clinical risk factors (MCRF) including age, height and weight on model performance. In this section, we detailly demonstrate our proposed MAResNet, which is shown in Fig. 1.

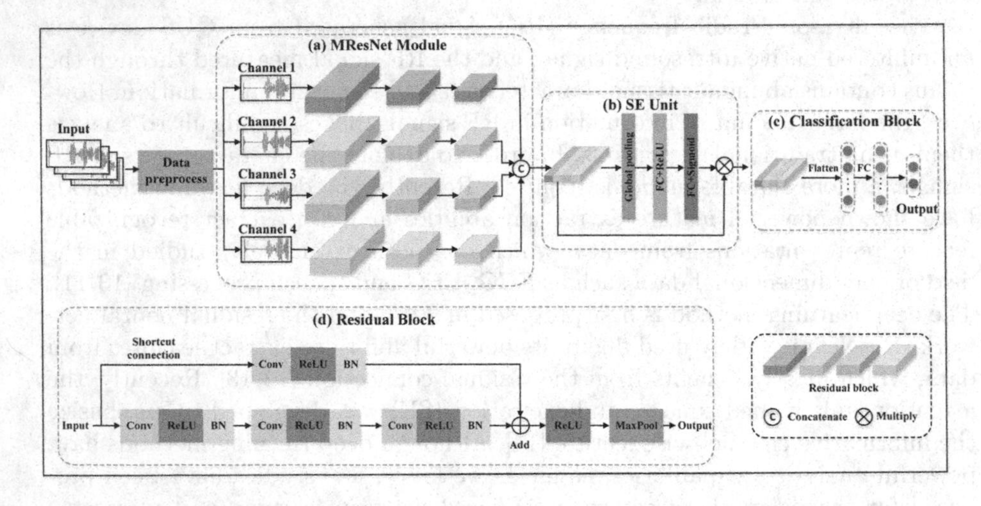

Fig. 1. Architecture of the proposed MAResNet, which consists of MResNet Module, SE Unit and Classification Block.

2.1 Multi-channel Residual Network Module

RF signals contain abundant temporal and spectral features which are difficult to extract manually. Therefore, as the feature extractor of this end-to-end network, the MResNet module extracts the features directly by the continuous residual blocks. As shown in Fig. 1(a), the RF signals source data of each channel is respectively input into the corresponding residual convolution path, forming the proposed multi-channel scheme. Each residual convolution path is connected to 3 residual blocks in turn. Figure 1(d) is the layout of the proposed Residual block, which includes 3 convolutional units. Each convolutional unit starts from a 1D convolutional layer with 8 filters, which generates a representation of RF signals. Then a Rectified Linear Unit (ReLU) is employed as the activation function to enhance the fitting ability of the model. Additionally, batch normalization operation is adopted in each unit to converge the model and alleviate the overfitting problem simultaneously. Specifically, the length of the 3 residual blocks convolution kernel of each channel is fixed to 8, 5 and 3 successively.

Different from the direct mapping in the shortcut connection of the original ResNet, a convolutional unit with 8 kernels of length 1 is added to the end of the successive convolutional units in this method. The residual connection enables the model to mitigate vanishing gradient effects. Then a max-pooling layer is employed to compress the feature vector by down-sampling.

For the 4 channels input, the input time series is represented by $r_{k,T} = (r_{k,1}, r_{k,2}, \ldots, r_{k,t})$, where the $r_{k,T}$ denotes the t-th time point of the k-th channel. For the data of the k-th channel, the output after the l-th residual block, that is, the input of the (l+1)-th residual block can be defined as:

$$X_{l+1,k} = F(X_{l,k}W^{c}_{l,k}) + X_{l,k}W^{r}_{l,k} \tag{1}$$

where $X_{l,k}$ is the input of the l-th residual block in the k-th channel, and when l=0, $X_{l,k}$ represents the input RF source data. $W^{r}_{l,k}$ and $W^{c}_{l,k}$ are the weights of shortcut connection and convolutional connection in the l-th residual block, respectively, and F represents the residual function. As a result, the MResNet module generates a set of RF data representations, which are then concatenated and fed into SE unit.

2.2 Squeeze-Excitation Attention Unit

Since the selection of features is crucial to the classification performance of osteoporosis, we add the SE unit for feature selection. After feature extraction through MResNet, the output feature vectors from all channels are concatenated in the channel direction and input into the SE unit. For the input feature map, the SE unit utilizes the compression-excitation mechanism to capture the correlation between channels and obtain the most discriminative features. Figure 1(b) depicts the structures of the SE unit. Specifically, in order to obtain the global distribution of channel feature responses, the "squeeze" operation firstly performs global-average pooling on the input feature maps to squeeze global information, and the output V_q calculated by global-average pooling can be expressed as:

$$V_q = \frac{1}{T}\sum_{t=1}^{T} X_c \tag{2}$$

where T is the length of the time series and X_c is the feature concatenating in the channel direction. After obtaining the global description features, the "excitation" operation is applied to obtain the correlation between feature channels, which generates weights for each feature channel to represent its importance. The "squeeze" operation consists of two fully-connection (FC) layer, where the ReLU function acts on the first FC layer and the Sigmoid function acts on the second. Then we apply the generated weights to the original input feature maps in the channel direction by multiplication to complete the feature recalibration, so as to obtain more discriminative features. After the channel-wise multiplying, the output V_e can be expressed as:

$$V_e = \epsilon(W_2\sigma(W_1V_q))X_c \tag{3}$$

where W_1 and W_2 are the connection weight parameters of the two fully connected layers in turn, and σ is the ReLU activation function, ϵ is the Sigmoid activation function. As a result, the channel-wise features can be fused and recalibrated.

2.3 Classification Block

Based on the selected channel-wise features, the classification module is designed to export the final decoding results. Specifically, the feature maps obtained above are first flatten to a feature vector. Then the vector is input into a FC layer with 512 neurons using the ReLU activation function, which follows a dropout layer with a random deactivation ratio of 0.5. It is denoted as:

$$f_n = W_nV_e + b_n \tag{4}$$

where f_n is the output of the n-th neuron, W_n and b_n is the connection weight and bias of the FC layer, respectively. Finally, the second FC layer is connected, with the Softmax function calculating the final output probabilities. It is noteworthy that the neurons number of the second FC layer is decided by whether the MCRF data is included. That is, when the MCRF is added, the neurons number increase from 10 to 13. We utilize the categorical cross-entropy as the loss function L, which can be defined as:

$$L = -\sum y_i \log f_i(x) \tag{5}$$

In Eq.(5), y_i is the true label corresponding to the i-th category, and $f_i(x)$ denotes the prediction probability generated by the model. Stochastic gradient descent (SGD) is used to update the model parameters and minimize the loss function, which aims to optimize the model performance.

3 Experimental Results

3.1 Datasets and Preprocessing

In this work, we use 274 cases of RF signal source data of radius to evaluate the proposed method, which is obtained from Sun Yat-sen Memorial Hospital, Sun Yat-sen University. QUS and DXA bone mineral density tests were performed on each subject on the same day and collected three times with an interval of more than 30 min. At the same time, information on MCRF including height, weight and age was collected for each subject. Based on the gold standard for the diagnosis of osteoporosis, DXA, the collected data can be divided into the following two categories: 181 subjects with normal bone mass and 93 subjects with osteoporosis, and the detailed data information can be found in Table 1.

Table 1. Detailed data information.

	Normal	Osteoporosis
Number	181	93
Age	58.88±10.85	67.18±9.52
Height	156.43±5.79	152.66±6.56
Weight	58.82±8.05	53.21±8.57

The equipemnt for data collection is Nanjing Kejin OSTEOKJ7000+ Ultrasound Bone Densitometer, which has two ultrasonic transmitters and two receivers, so it can simultaneously collect four channels of RF signals. A single channel outputs 105 frames of RF signals about 20 s, and each frame has 1024 time points. In this paper, we intercept the effectively transmitted signal from each frame, that is, the data of 725 acquisition time points, and then convert the intercepted data into a value with an amplitude in the range of 0–255. Simultaneously, we perform Butterworth low pass filtering on the data for denoising. For each subject, we utilize continuously temporal data of 725 time points so that the length of data from a channel of each subject is 228375.

3.2 Experiment Setup

The dataset is randomly divided into training set and test set, which contains 234 and 40 subjects, respectively. In order to mitigate the impact of data distribution, all the groups had almost the same category ratio. The detection results of DXA are used as true labels. We use the training set data to train the model to ensure that the model has the predictive ability. The experiments are carried out on a workstation using the deep learning framework TensorFlow with a single NVIDIA GPU.

We compare the traditional method using SOS with the proposed method. Simultaneously, in order to verify the superiority of the performance of the proposed model, we use machine learning methods SVM and Random Forest, deep learning methods LSTM [15], MobileNet [16] and CNN models to make comparisons, and discuss the effect of adding the MCRF of the subjects on the proposed model. Specifically, the CNN is connected by 5 simple 1D convolution layers, and each convolution layer has 8 convolution kernels with a size of 5 with the ReLU activation function. In the experiments, classification accuracy (ACC), specificity (SPE), sensitivity (SEN), F1-score (F1), area under curve (AUC) and

Kappa are utilized to evaluate the proposed MAResNet. In addition, all deep learning models are optimized using SGD optimization algorithm, and the initial learning rate is 0.0001. The batch size is set to 16, and the number of epochs is 200.

3.3 Results

In this paper, we compare the classification results of conventional QUS methods using SOS, SVM, Random Fore st, LSTM, MobileNet and CNN of each subject with the proposed MAResNet, which is summarized by Table 2. From Table 2, we can learn that the overall accuracy based on SOS is 0.679, which is lower than the accuracy of 0.786 for RF signals using MAResNet. Meanwhile, the SVM, Random Forest, LSTM, MobileNet and CNN get the accuracy of 0.690, 0.694, 0.756, 0.743 and 0.767, respectively, which is lower than the proposed MAResNet, indicateing that MAResNet has a better performance. Specifically, when adding MCRF to the proposed model, such as age, height and weight, the MAResNet with MCRF achieves the best accuracy of 0.818 and gets the optimal overall performance. Furthermore, our method yields F1-score of 0.700 and SEN of 0.623, which are the best among these methods. Although our method decreases the SPE slightly, it improves the SEN greatly, which is of great significance for the correct diagnosis of osteoporosis patients.

Table 2. Osteoporosis classification performance using different methods.

Method	ACC	SPE	SEN	F1	AUC	Kappa
SVM	0.690	**0.992**	0.117	0.203	0.554	0.136
Random Forest	0.694	0.967	0.176	0.278	0.572	0.174
SOS	0.679	0.791	0.457	0.488	0.624	0.343
LSTM	0.756	0.951	0.449	0.575	0.701	0.227
MobileNet	0.743	0.949	0.357	0.472	0.604	0.445
CNN	0.767	0.955	0.417	0.552	0.695	0.419
MAResNet	0.786	0.927	0.524	0.623	0.750	0.487
MAResNet+MCRF	**0.818**	0.923	**0.623**	**0.700**	**0.824**	**0.575**

where the bold values indicate the best results.

Additionally, Fig. 2 shows the ROC and AUC of different diagnostic methods for osteoporosis diagnosis. The AUC of SOS and other comparison models is lower than the AUC of MAResNet, which is 0.750. The AUC is significantly improved when adding MCRF to the MAResNet, which increases to 0.824. It is around 0.2 higher than the conventional QUS method using SOS. Figure 3 shows the confusion matrix of SOS and all the models this paper adopts, where 0 denotes osteoporosis and 1 denotes normal. It can be seen from the confusion matrix

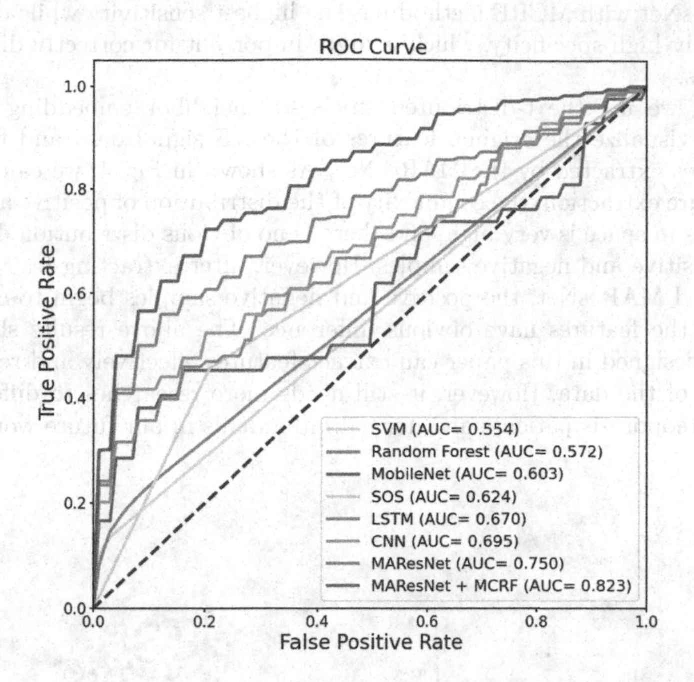

Fig. 2. ROC curve of different methods.

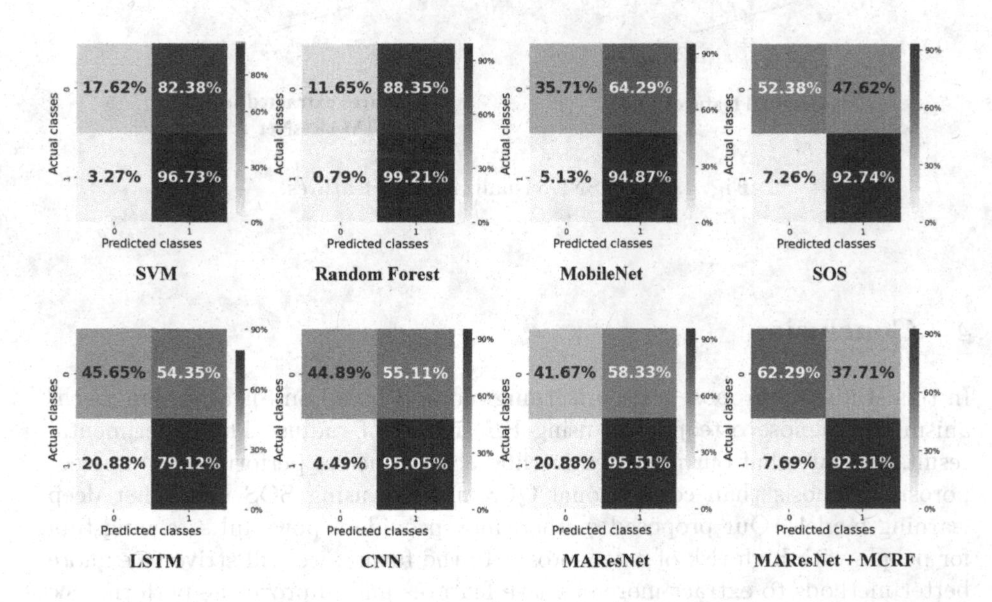

Fig. 3. The confusion matrix on the dataset.

that MAResNet with MCRF method has the highest sensitivity while obtaining the relatively high specificity, which is quite important for correctly diagnosing osteoporosis.

Besides, we use the t-distributed stochastic neighbor embedding (t-SNE) method to visualize the original features of the RF signal data and the high-level features extracted by the MAResNet. As shown in Fig. 4, we can see that before feature extraction, the complexity of the distribution of positive and negative samples in space is very high, and there is no obvious distribution difference between positive and negative samples. However, after extracting features with the proposed MAResNet, the positive and negative samples begin to cluster in space, and the features have obvious difference. The above results show that the model designed in this paper can extract features effectively and reduce the complexity of the data. However, it still needs more researches to differentiate between osteoporosis patients and normal individuals in our future work.

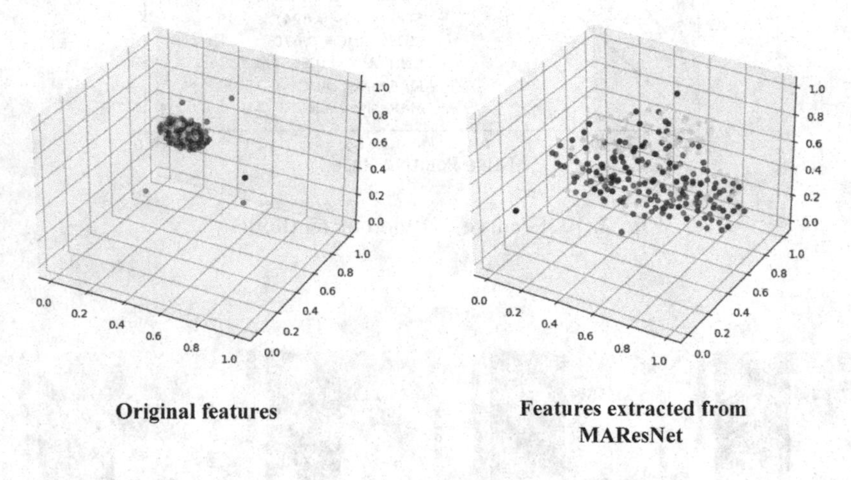

Fig. 4. The t-SNE visualization of features.

4 Conclusion

In this study, we propose a deep learning method based on SE attention mechanism to diagnose osteoporosis using RF signals of radius. The experimental results indicate that our proposed method achieve better performance on osteoporosis diagnosis than conventional QUS method using SOS and other deep learning models. Our proposed method may provide a powerful screening tool for people with high risk of osteoporosis. In the future, we will strive to explore better methods to extract more effective features and improve the performance of osteoporosis diagnosis based on RF signals.

Acknowledgements. This study was approved by the Sun Yat-sen Memorial Hospital Ethics Board (No: SYSEC-KY-KS-2019-159) and satisfied the criteria of the World Medical Association Declaration of Helsinki-Ethical Principles for Medical Research.

References

1. Rachner, T.D., Khosla, S., Hofbauer, L.C.: Osteoporosis: now and the future. Lancet **377**(9773), 1276–1287 (2011)
2. Link, T.M., Kazakia, G.: Update on imaging-based measurement of bone mineral density and quality. Curr. Rheumatol. Rep. **22**(5), 1–11 (2020). https://doi.org/10.1007/s11926-020-00892-w
3. Fuggle, N.R., Curtis, E.M., Ward, K.A., Harvey, N.C., Dennison, E.M., Cooper, C.: Fracture prediction, imaging and screening in osteoporosis. Nat. Rev. Endocrinol. **15**(9), 535–547 (2019)
4. Watts, N.B.: The fracture risk assessment tool (frax(r)): applications in clinical practice. J Womens Health (Larchmt) **20**(4), 525–531 (2011)
5. Langton, C., Palmer, S., Porter, R.: The measurement of broadband ultrasonic attenuation in cancellous bone. Eng. Med. **13**(2), 89–91 (1984)
6. Raef, H., Al-Bugami, M., Balharith, S., Moawad, M.: Updated recommendations for the diagnosis and management of osteoporosis: a local perspective. Ann. Saudi Med. **31**(2), 111–128 (2011)
7. Fu, Y., Li, C., Luo, W., Chen, Z., Liu, Z., Ding, Y.: Fragility fracture discriminative ability of radius quantitative ultrasound: a systematic review and meta-analysis. Osteoporos. Int. **32**, 1–16 (2020). https://doi.org/10.1007/s00198-020-05559-x
8. Guyon, I., Elisseeff, A.: An introduction to variable and feature selection. J. Mach. Learn. Res. **3**, 1157–1182 (2003)
9. Nayak, S., et al.: Meta-analysis: accuracy of quantitative ultrasound for identifying patients with osteoporosis. Ann. Intern. Med. **144**(11), 832–841 (2006)
10. Somani, S., Adam, J.R., Felix, R., Shan, Z., Akhil, V., Fayzan, C.: Deep learning and the electrocardiogram: review of the current state-of-the-art. EP Europace **23**(8), 1179–1191 (2021)
11. Ismail Fawaz, H., Forestier, G., Weber, J., Idoumghar, L., Muller, P.-A.: Deep learning for time series classification: a review. Data Min. Knowl. Discovery **33**(4), 917–963 (2019)
12. He, K., Zhang, X., Ren, S., Sun, J.: Deep residual learning for image recognition. In: Proceedings of the IEEE Conference on Computer Vision and Pattern Recognition, Nevada, pp. 770–778 (2016)
13. He, F., Liu, T., Tao, D.: Why resnet works? residuals generalize. IEEE Trans. Neural Netw. Learn. syst. **31**(12), 5349–5362 (2020)
14. Hu, J., Shen, L., Sun, G.: Squeeze-and-excitation networks. In: Proceedings of the IEEE Conference on Computer Vision and Pattern Recognition, Utah, pp. 7132–7141 (2018)
15. Hochreiter, S., Schmidhuber, J.: Long short-term memory. Neural Comput. **9**(8), 1735–1780 (1997). https://doi.org/10.1007/978-3-642-24797-2_4
16. Howard, A.G., Zhu, M., Chen, B., Kalenichenko, D., Wang, W., Weyand, T.: Mobilenets: efficient convolutional neural networks for mobile vision applications. arXiv preprint. arXiv:1704.04861 (2017)

Machine Learning Based Approach for Motion Detection and Estimation in Routinely Acquired Low Resolution Near Infrared Fluorescence Optical Imaging

Lukas Zerweck[1,3(✉)], Stefan Wesarg[2,3], Jörn Kohlhammer[2,3], and Michaela Köhm[1,3,4]

[1] Fraunhofer Institute for Translational Medicine and Pharmacology ITMP, Frankfurt am Main, Germany
lukas.zerweck@itmp.fraunhofer.de
[2] Fraunhofer Institute for Computer Graphics Research IGD, Darmstadt, Germany
[3] Fraunhofer Cluster of Excellence Immune-Mediated Diseases CIMD, Frankfurt am Main, Germany
[4] Division of Rheumatology, Goethe-University Frankfurt, Frankfurt am Main, Germany

Abstract. Near infrared fluorescence optical imaging (NIR-FOI) visualises the vascular perfusion of the investigated anatomical structure. Even though there has been a lot of medical research in the field to detect joint inflammation utilising NIR-FOI, an objective machine learning based evaluation method of the image data has not been developed, yet.

The measured NIR-FOI data consists of two spatial dimensions (image pixel) and one temporal dimension. To assess the distribution process an understanding of the hands' locations is essential. However, random motion changes the positioning, which requires re-segmentation. The goal of this work is to identify the time points (frames) and severity of motion in the previously measured image stack. Due to properties of the NIR-FOI, each data set is split into two phases: Before and after full illumination of the hands. For each phase, an independent model is trained to evaluate the severity and time point of possible motion.

The model for the first phase achieves a precision of 20.78 % and a recall of 69.57 %, while the model for the second phase reaches a precision of 67.71 % and a recall of 98.49 % to detect non-negligible motion. Despite low precision, both models can be considered a success, contemplating the high heterogeneity, self-illumination and real-life consequences of a low precision value, which only affects computation time.

Our general goal is to achieve a robust and early detection of psoriatic arthritis, to increase quality of life while decreasing treatment costs. The presented work plays a key role in this research, especially increasing robustness of the final evaluation pipeline.

Y. Chen et al. (Eds.): CLIP 2022, LNCS 13746, pp. 22–31, 2023.
https://doi.org/10.1007/978-3-031-23179-7_3

Keywords: Fluorescence optical imaging · Motion detection · Self-illuminated object detection

1 Introduction and Motivation

Different types of arthritis can lead to structural damage in the joints. An early and correct diagnosis is crucial to prevent joint damage and keep full functionality [4,7]. Today, arthritis is diagnosed via clinical examination of tender and swollen joints or additionally, exploiting imaging modalities such as ultrasound or MRI [6,8]. One relatively new imaging modality, which might be able to detect clinical psoriatic arthritis (PsA) is near infrared fluorescence optical imaging (NIR-FOI) [13]. Being less expensive than MRI and less assessor dependent than ultrasound, this imaging modality could provide valuable insights for the early detection of PsA.

NIR-FOI is a near infrared imaging modality, in which the colour agent indocyanine green (ICG) is administered to the patient [13]. During the 6 min after injection the distribution of the ICG in the hands is detected by taking a series of 360 images (1 image per second). In the following the term *data set* refers to one image stack of 360 images. Three exemplary images are visualised in Fig. 1. This leads to a 3-dimensional data space (two spatial dimensions x, y and one temporal dimension t). In accordance to previous work, we hypothesise that the shape of the ICG distribution enables to classify the joints in the hands into arthritis affected and unaffected [13]. In order to describe the distribution process, both hands are segmented into 33 areas corresponding to anatomical structures such as joints and fingers (the segmentation is inspired by [5,10]). The time series of these 33 areas can then be investigated to evaluate their health status. All areas need to be identified for all images in the stack in order to extract these time series. The motion detection is one pre-processing step to correctly identify each area in every slice of the image stack considering possible motion of the patient.

The segmentation is computed for one reference image by a customised fully convolution neural network based on an U-Net architecture [12]. This CNN is trained from scratch with labelled NIR-FOI data utilising deep learning (an U-Net result is shown in Fig. 1d). Then it is projected to the remaining images in the stack. Using one reference segmentation mask instead of segmenting every individual image in the stack, is mainly caused by the self-illumination process of the hands (a detailed description of the process is given in Sect. 2.3). The time and order in which the parts of the hands are illuminating are highly dependent on the data set. The amount of labelled data necessary to train a robust neural network segmenting each image for this phase is not available.

A second reason to compute one reference segmentation mask and project it to the remaining image stack is the small amount of computations. As mentioned before, the presented work is part of a project to detect PsA in NIR-FOI. Thus, the final evaluation pipeline, including the motion detection, should run in a feasible time on hospital work stations. These are most often low-performance GPU-free machines, encouraging classic computer vision techniques.

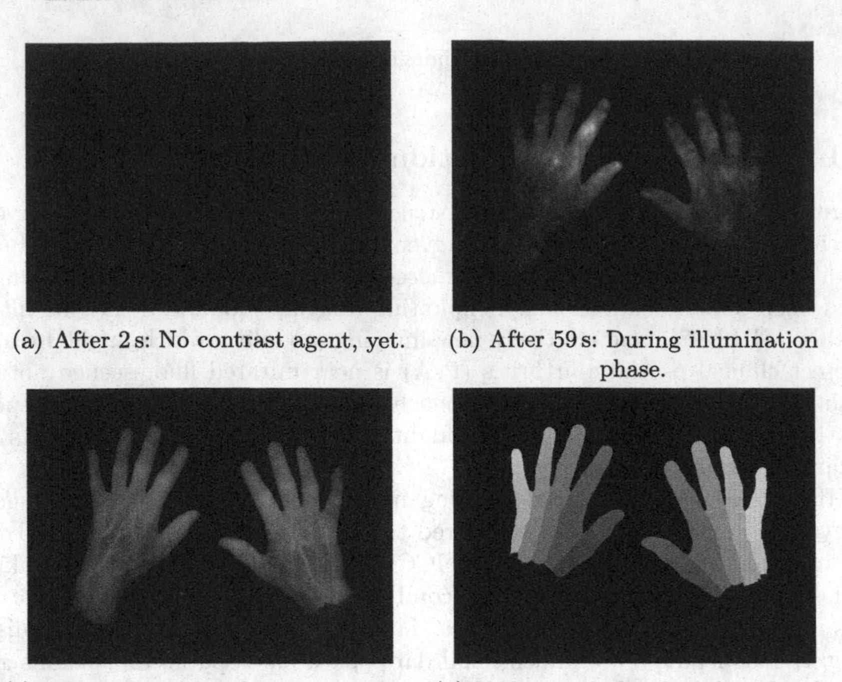

(a) After 2 s: No contrast agent, yet.

(b) After 59 s: During illumination phase.

(c) After 250 s: After full illumination. Flush out phase.

(d) U-Net result for the left and right hand.

Fig. 1. (a) - (c): Three images at different time points. The image stack is contrast-enhanced by histogram stretching using the minimal and maximal value of the whole image stack as references. (d): Visualisation of the segmentation result.

However, using one fixed mask for all images assumes that the hands are completely still for 6 min, which is rarely the case. Therefore, the time points at which the hands are changing position must be identified and the segmentation mask updated correspondingly.

In this work, we suggest a pipeline to detect motion artefacts and their specific time points (frame) in NIR-FOI data sets based on classic computer vision techniques as well as machine learning models. The pipeline has been developed and evaluated on clinical images, with the same structure and patient distribution as routinely acquired image data.

2 Background

2.1 Related Work

NIR-FOI as a diagnostic tool for arthritis diagnosis has been the subject of ongoing research for roughly a decade. Nonetheless, there were only a few early attempts to automatically evaluate the data [3,9], none of which tackled the issue of motion artefacts. Thus, the medical and the computer vision background are discussed separately.

Medical Work. The sensitivity and specificity of NIR-FOI in comparison to other imaging modalities, such as MRI and ultrasound as well as to the medical investigation have been analysed in detail (e.g. in [8,13]). All these studies show the potential of NIR-FOI in the diagnosis of arthritis, though the semi-quantitative evaluation method of the images (the data sets are evaluated by a medical professional) motivate an automated and objective approach.

Computer Vision Background of Motion Detection. In images or volumes without a temporal component, such as MRI or CAT scans, motion artefacts lead to distorted or blurred objects. These need to be detected and corrected within the spatial dimensions. However, the NIR-FOI data space contains one temporal dimension and thus, motion does not distort or blur the object of interest but changes the location necessitating a re-segmentation. Due to the different nature of the data, the wide range of approaches to detect and remove motion artefacts within MRI and CAT scans cannot be applied.

Caused by the temporal dimension, detecting motion in the NIR-FOI data is similar to detect motion in videos, such as camera feeds. However, most used approaches from less complex (such as image differentiation) to more advanced algorithms (such as optical flow [1]) do not work on the NIR-FOI data. This is mainly caused by the rapidly changing illumination, especially during the illumination phase (e.g. stable illumination is one of the main conditions to use optical flow). Another common approach is using key point detection and -tracking models to detect motion. This approach might work for parts of the data (after full illumination of the hands), though pre-trained models do not achieve a satisfying result especially over consecutive images. The change of positioning of key points referring to the same anatomical structure in consecutive images caused by noise or motion are in the same magnitude. Additionally, no labelled data is available to fine tune existing models.

2.2 Participants

122 data sets were used to investigate the motion artefacts. Out of these, 62 data sets were acquired in a study investigating early psoriatic arthritis using NIR-FOI as one modality. The remaining 60 data sets where recorded for a study investigating systemic sclerosis using NIR-FOI as imaging modality. A signed consent to the corresponding study protocol and agreement to the usage of their data for research purposes was provided by all participants, who were all fully capable of giving informed consent. Both studies fulfilled Good Clinical Practices Guidelines and all medical procedures were performed according to the study protocol. The protocols of both studies have been approved by the responsible ethics committee.

2.3 Data

As mentioned in Sect. 1 the acquired data consists of two spatial dimensions x and y referring to the pixel indices in the images and one temporal dimension

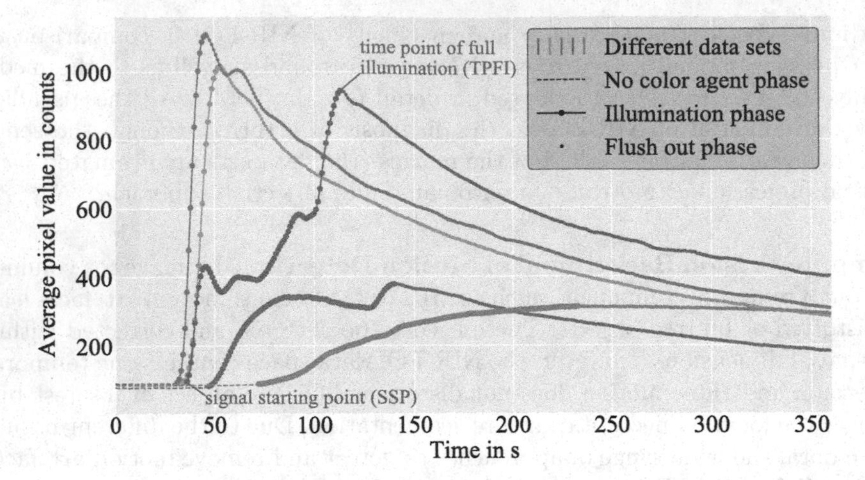

Fig. 2. Five average time line examples, showing the diverse shapes of the illumination process.

t corresponding to the consecutive image acquisition. In the beginning of the 360 images the ICG has not reached the hands yet and therefore the images are only containing noise (see Fig. 1a). After an undefined time period, varying for each data set, the colour agent reaches the hands (signal starting point SSP) and parts of the hands are starting to be self-illuminated[1] (see Fig. 1b). Even though there are models describing the illumination process [6], the hands of every person illuminate in different shapes and speeds. After the hands are fully illuminated (time point of full illumination TPFI), the flush out phase of the colour agent starts (see Fig. 1c). The data sets do not only differ in illumination speed and shape but also in overall brightness. In Fig. 2 five exemplary time series are visualised and the individual phases and one exemplary SSD and TPFI are marked. In order to extract these time series, the average count for each frame (x, y dimensions) is calculated.

All data sets were acquired with the same machine to reduce variability. The data acquisition process was already described in detail in previous work [8,10,13].

3 Method

As mentioned in Sect. 2.3 the illumination process can be split into the phase before and after full illumination (FI) of the hands. Since the challenges of detecting motion differ for these two phases, two separate algorithms are developed.

For both cases, the final classification of each image as motionless or motion affected is performed by a support vector machine (SVM) [2]. In order to train

[1] The term self-illumination refers to the ICG emitted light being the only measured light source. Visibility, brightness etc. depend on the investigated hands' conditions.

these models, each image is labelled as no motion, negligible motion and non-negligible motion (three classes), in comparison to each previous image. When evaluating the model's performance the no motion and negligible motion class are merged, since images of both classes have no impact on the area time series (see Sect. 1). The labelling is based on human level perception.

3.1 Before FI

After the TPFI is determined by calculating the average count for each image in the image stack (compare Sect. 2.3) the binary mask for this image is calculated (reference mask). Additionally, the extracted time series is used to calculate the SSP. All described processes in this subchapter refer to the time period after the SSP and before the TPFI $t_{\mathrm{SSP}\sim\mathrm{TPFI}}$ (one example of the SSP and TPFI is given in Fig. 2).

The motion detection of this time period can be split into two steps. Firstly, the existence of motion in general is evaluated. If motion is detected, a second step evaluating the time point and severity of the motion is carried out.

In order to check if the hands are moved at any time point during $t_{\mathrm{SSP}\sim\mathrm{TPFI}}$, firstly a binary mask is computed (foreground mask). This mask includes all pixels, which are part of the hands at any given time point during $t_{\mathrm{SSP}\sim\mathrm{TPFI}}$. The mask is based on a differentiation image, calculated by firstly subtracting the background time series from each pixel's time series and secondly, choosing the maximal difference as pixel value. The background time series is based on the average count of small regions in the four image corners.

After cropping the image stack, foreground and reference mask to the bounding box of the foreground mask ($w_{\mathrm{fg}} \cdot h_{\mathrm{fg}}$) the bottom left and bottom right area of each image in the stack as well as the two masks are set to zero. These areas contain the wrist and lower arm signals and are of little interest. Removing these areas decreases the amount of unwanted signal drastically.

Now, the overlay of the two masks is calculated using the Intercept-over-Union (IoU) score [11]. If the score exceeds 98.5 % no motion is detected and the whole time period before reaching FI is considered motionless. This boundary value has been defined after extensive testing and is purely empirical, leading to the best observed results.

In cases which do not reach an overlap of 98.5 % or more, further analysis steps are carried out to evaluate the time points of motion. Firstly, the difference between each image and its preceding image is calculated (difference image stack). To evaluate which pixels in this stack are part of a possible motion, a boundary map is computed based on the median along t. If the boundary is exceeded, the pixel is considered a possible motion. This method generates some salt-and-pepper noise, which is reduced by a median filter. As a final preparation step, two values per image are computed: The number of connected foreground areas is counted and the density of foreground pixels $\frac{w_{\mathrm{fg}} \cdot h_{\mathrm{fg}}}{\#\ \mathrm{foreground\ pixel}}$ is calculated. These two numbers across multiple data sets are used to train a SVM to classify each image into one of the three classes.

3.2 After FI

All described processes in this Subsection refer to the time period between the calculated TPFI (see Fig. 2) mentioned in the previous section and the end of the data set. The overall idea of determining a motion in comparison to the previous image is based on the computation of a binary mask per image and the subtraction from the binary mask of the previous image. However, regulatory measures need to be included in the process to eliminate overlaying effects, such as movements of irrelevant areas and noise.

In a first step, an individual binary mask for each image is calculated. Thus, each image is segmented into fore- (hand regions) and background. During this process, the maximal bounding box, including all kind of movements, is determined. As mentioned before, the wrist and lower arm regions are of little interest and thus, are removed from all pictures and masks.

Since the hands do not have clear edges, the determined binary masks fluctuate along the temporal dimension t in the transition area from fore- to background (hand edges). To reduce the impact of these fluctuations, a noise map is defined, based on the pixel-wise alternation between fore- and background. After the difference mask stack (DMS) is calculated by subtracting each consecutive pair of masks from each other, the pixels defined in the noise map are set to zero in the whole DMS, followed by the removal of small holes and - areas. The DMS now contains only large regions of change between two consecutive images not considering the wrists and lower arm regions. For each movement mask in the DMS, the amount of foreground pixels is counted and the average area size calculated. This leads to two values per image for each data set, which are used to train a SVM to classify each image into one of the three classes.

4 Results

All described methods and calculations were implemented using Python 3.8, with the following setup: Tensorflow 2.3.0, Tensorflow.keras 2.4.0, Sklearn 0.24.2 and OpenCV 4.0.1. In the following the term *data point* refers to one frame.

For the time period before FI, 7685 data points are available, with 7499 labelled as no motion, 100 labelled as negligible and 76 labelled as non-negligible motion. The data set is split with a ratio of 70 % training data and 30 % test data, which leads to 5249 no motion, 77 negligible and 53 non-negligible motion data points in the training data set. Accordingly 2250 no motion, 33 negligible and 23 non-negligible motion samples are in the test data set.

For the time period after FI 31 593 data points are available, with 30 894 labelled as no motion, 480 labelled as negligible and 219 as non-negligible motion. The data set is also split with a ratio of 70 % training data and 30 % test data, which leads to 21 625 no motion, 336 negligible and 153 non-negligible motion data points in the training data set. Accordingly, 9269 no motion, 144 negligible and 66 non-negligible motion samples are in the test data set.

In order to train the SVMs, in both cases data preparation steps are performed. Firstly, the training data set is shuffled, followed by a normalising step

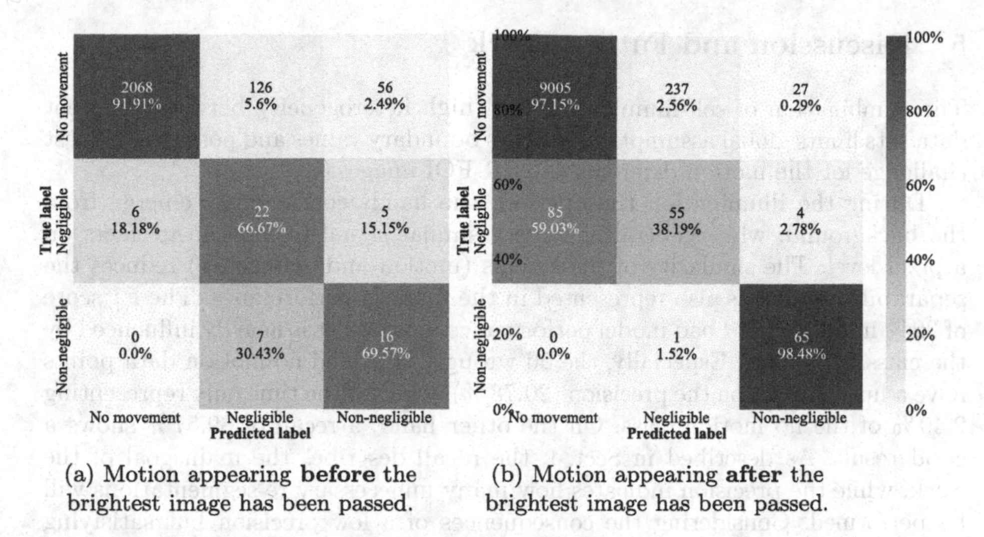

(a) Motion appearing **before** the brightest image has been passed.

(b) Motion appearing **after** the brightest image has been passed.

Fig. 3. Confusion matrices for the performances of the ML models to discriminate between no, negligible and non-negligible motions.

using the z-score as metric (setting mean to zero and variance to one). Finally, the impact of the highly unbalanced class sizes during the training process is removed by weighting each sample by the inverse class size (e.g. samples of the no motion class in the data set after FI are weighted with a factor of $\frac{1}{30894}$). To test the trained model with the test data set, each data point is scaled based on the computed mean and variance of the training data set (z-score).

The classification results are visualised in Fig. 3. However, the main goal of this work is to detect non-negligible motion and thus, this class is described in more detail. For the time period before FI out of the 23 labelled data points 16 are classified correctly, which amounts to a recall of 69.57 %. From the classes no motion and negligible motion, 61 data points are falsely classified as non-negligible motion, which leads to a precision of 20.78 %. The computed recall and precision values result in a F1 score of 32 %.

In the period after FI, out of 66 non-negligible motion data points 65 are classified correctly, which results in a recall of 98.49 %. Furthermore, 31 data points are falsely classified as non-negligible, which amounts to a precision of 67.71 %. These values lead to a F1 score of 80.25 %.

In the work at hand, the recall defines how many non-negligible motions are detected and thus, has a direct impact on the evaluation of the segmented hand areas. The recall for both models is satisfying with one being nearly perfect. These values represent the main goal of the work. The precision indicates how many unnecessary re-segmentations will be performed and therefore, represents the second objective of the work. However, it does not have a direct impact on the evaluation result of the hand areas and only increases the calculation time. Thus, a high precision is aspired but less important than a high recall.

5 Discussion and Future Work

The combination of self-illumination and high heterogeneity between different data sets limits global assumptions such as boundary values and poses the biggest challenge for the motion detection in NIR-FOI images.

During the illumination time period, the hands continuously emerge from the background, while generating a very similar signal to motion artefacts on a pixel level. The similarity of the signals (motion and emergence) reduces the separability, which is also represented in the model's performance. The F1 score of 32 % implies a very bad model performance, however it is heavily influenced by the class imbalance. Especially, the 56 wrongly classified no motion data points have a huge impact on the precision (20.78 %), while at the time only representing 2.49 % of the no motion class. On the other hand, a recall of 69.57 % shows a good result. As described in Sect. 4, the recall describes the main goal of the work, while the precision indicates how many unnecessary re-segmentations will be performed. Considering the consequences of a low precision but satisfying recall value, the model at hand can be considered mainly successful.

In the second time period (after FI) the hands are already fully visible and thus, motion is not overlaid by emerging parts of the hands. This has a positive effect on the separability, which is also represented by the model's performance. A recall of 98.49 % indicates that almost all non-negligible motions have been identified. Even though a precision of 67.71 % is already a satisfying result, it is again highly influenced by the huge class imbalance. Only 0.29 % of the no motion class have been misclassified as non-negligible motion while accounting for 27 data points. This amounts to 41 % of the total number of non-negligible motion samples (66). Considering the consequences of a lower precision and higher recall value, the model of this phase can be considered well-working.

In the presented work one part of the pre-processing pipeline to investigate PsA in NIR-FOI is given. Based on the achieved results, motion can be identified and its effects compensated: An important step towards disease diagnosis.

In the future, a neural network could replace the SVM to achieve better results on the classification into the three classes. Additionally, other pre-processing steps need to be included to enable a PsA diagnosis. These include, among other things, motion detection of slow and steady movements, ambient light identification and an understanding of the heterogeneous ICG distribution process among different patients. After the data preparation is completed, an automated image classification can be developed.

Acknowledgements. We thank Ulf Henkemeier and team for the data acquisition. Additionally, we thank Andreas Wirtz, Raaghav Radhakrishnan and Phuong-Ha Nguyen for valuable discussions.

References

1. Beauchemin, S.S., Barron, J.L.: The computation of optical flow. ACM Comput. Surv. **27**(3), 433–466 (1995). https://doi.org/10.1145/212094.212141
2. Cortes, C., Vapnik, V.: Support-vector networks. Mach. Learn. **20**(3), 273–297 (1995). https://doi.org/10.1007/bf00994018
3. Dziekan, T., et al.: Detection of rheumatoid arthritis by evaluation of normalized variances of fluorescence time correlation functions. J. Biomed. Opt. **16**(7), 076015 (2011). https://doi.org/10.1117/1.3599958
4. Finckh, A., Liang, M.H., van Herckenrode, C.M., de Pablo, P.: Long-term impact of early treatment on radiographic progression in rheumatoid arthritis: a meta-analysis. Arthritis Care Res. **55**(6), 864–872 (2006). https://doi.org/10.1002/art.22353
5. Friedrich, S., et al.: Disturbed microcirculation in the hands of patients with systemic sclerosis detected by fluorescence optical imaging: a pilot study. Arthritis Res. Ther. **19**(1), 1–13 (2017). https://doi.org/10.1186/s13075-017-1300-6
6. Glimm, A.M., Werner, S.G., Burmester, G.R., Backhaus, M., Ohrndorf, S.: Analysis of distribution and severity of inflammation in patients with osteoarthitis compared to rheumatoid arthritis by ICG-enhanced fluorescence optical imaging and musculoskeletal ultrasound: a pilot study. Ann. Rheum. Dis. **75**(3), 566–570 (2015). https://doi.org/10.1136/annrheumdis-2015-207345
7. Haroon, M., Gallagher, P., FitzGerald, O.: Diagnostic delay of more than 6 months contributes to poor radiographic and functional outcome in psoriatic arthritis. Ann. Rheum. Dis. **74**(6), 1045–1050 (2014). https://doi.org/10.1136/annrheumdis-2013-204858
8. Hirano, F.: Comparison of fluorescence optical imaging, ultrasonography and clinical examination with magnetic resonance imaging as a reference in active rheumatoid arthritis patients. Immunol. Med. **41**(2), 75–81 (2018). https://doi.org/10.1080/13497413.2018.1481578
9. Mohajerani, P., Meier, R., Noël, P.B., Rummeny, E.J., Ntziachristos, V.: Spatiotemporal analysis for indocyanine green-aided imaging of rheumatoid arthritis in hand joints. J. Biomed. Optics **18**(9), 097004 (2013). https://doi.org/10.1117/1.jbo.18.9.097004
10. Pfeil, A., et al.: The application of fluorescence optical imaging in systemic sclerosis. Biomed. Res. Int. **2015**, 1–6 (2015). https://doi.org/10.1155/2015/658710
11. Rezatofighi, H., Tsoi, N., Gwak, J., Sadeghian, A., Reid, I., Savarese, S.: Generalized intersection over union: a metric and a loss for bounding box regression. In: 2019 IEEE/CVF Conference on Computer Vision and Pattern Recognition (CVPR). IEEE (2019). https://doi.org/10.1109/cvpr.2019.00075
12. Ronneberger, O., Fischer, P., Brox, T.: U-Net: convolutional networks for biomedical image segmentation (2015). https://doi.org/10.48550/ARXIV.1505.04597
13. Werner, S.G., et al.: Indocyanine green-enhanced fluorescence optical imaging in patients with early and very early arthritis: a comparative study with magnetic resonance imaging. Arthritis Rheum. **65**(12), 3036–3044 (2013). https://doi.org/10.1002/art.38175

Automatic Landmark Identification on IntraOralScans

Baptiste Baquero[1,9](✉), Maxime Gillot[1,9], Lucia Cevidanes[1], Najla Al Turkestani[1,5], Marcela Gurgel[1], Mathieu Leclercq[4,9], Jonas Bianchi[1,3], Marilia Yatabe[1], Antonio Ruellas[1,2], Camila Massaro[8], Aron Aliaga[1], Maria Antonia Alvarez Castrillon[6], Diego Rey[6], Juan Fernando Aristizabal[7], and Juan Carlos Prieto[4]

[1] University of Michigan, Michigan, USA
baptistebaquero@gmail.com
[2] Federal University of Rio de Janeiro, Rio de Janeiro, Brazil
[3] University of the Pacific, San Francisco, USA
[4] University of North Carolina, Chapel Hill, USA
[5] King Abdulaziz University, Jeddah, Saudi Arabia
[6] CES University, Medellín, Colombia
[7] University of Valle, Cali, Colombia
[8] Federal University of Goiás, Goiânia, Brazil
[9] CPE Lyon, Lyon, France

Abstract. With the advent of 3D printing and additive manufacturing of dental devices, IntraOral scanners (IOS) have gained wide adoption in dental practices and allowed for efficient workflows in clinical settings. Accurate automatic identification of dental landmarks in IOS is required to aid dental researchers and clinicians to plan and assess tooth position for crown restorations, orthodontics movements, and/or implant dentistry. In this paper, we present a new algorithm for Automatic Landmark Identification on IntraOralScans (ALIIOS), that combines image processing, image segmentation, and machine learning approaches to automatically and accurately identify commonly used landmarks on IOSs. Four hundred and five digital dental models were pre-processed by 3 clinician experts to manually annotate 5 landmarks on each dental crown in the upper and lower arches. Our approach uses the PyTorch3D rendering engine to capture 2D views of the dental arches from different viewpoints as well as the target 3D patches at the location of the landmarks. The ALIIOS algorithm synthesizes these 3D patches with a U-Net and allows accurate placement of the landmarks on the surface of each dental crown. Our results, after cross-validation, show an average distance error between the prediction and the clinicians' landmarks of 0.43 ± 0.28 mm and 0.45 ± 0.28 mm for respectively lower and upper occlusal landmarks, and 0.62 ± 0.28 mm for lower and upper cervical landmarks. There was on average a 5% error of landmarks more than 1.5 mm away from the clinicians' landmarks, due to errors in landmark nomenclature or improper segmentation. In conclusion, we present and validate a novel algorithm for accurate automated landmark identification on intraoral scans to increase efficiency and facilitate quantitative assessments in clinical practice.

Y. Chen et al. (Eds.): CLIP 2022, LNCS 13746, pp. 32–42, 2023.
https://doi.org/10.1007/978-3-031-23179-7_4

Keywords: Deep learning · Automatic landmark identification · Digital dental model

1 Introduction

Digital dental models are obtained by Intraoral scans (IOS are widely used in dentistry). Even if many practices still lack this technology, conventional plaster models are now digitized as services provided by laboratories, to plan the proper placement of the dental crowns, tooth movement [3], fabrication of dental restorations [2], monitoring and maintaining periodontal health, attaining stable treatment outcomes, and the occlusal function [11]. IOSs are detailed 3D surface mesh models of the upper and lower dentition that allow clinicians to accurately evaluate the clinical crown position in three dimensions without radiation exposure to the patient [1]. Time efficiency increased patient comfort, and data fusion options within a computer-aided design and manufacturing technologies increasingly used in dentistry are among the multiple advantages of IOS systems [5]. Given that intraoral scanning and digitization of tooth geometries is a fundamental step in the dental digital workflow, the accuracy of measurements in IOS must be evaluated critically. Dentists need to segment each tooth in the IOS and annotate the corresponding anatomical landmarks to analyze, rearrange and/or restore tooth position. Manual performance of these tasks is time-consuming and prone to inconsistency. There is a clinical need to develop fully automatic methods instead of manual operation. The development of an artificial intelligence tool for landmark localization of dental crown surfaces is challenging, mainly due to variability of the anatomical structures of different teeth, abnormal, disarranged, and/or missing teeth for some patients. Compared with the individual tooth segmentation and labeling, the localization of anatomical landmarks is typically more sensitive to the variable shape appearance of each patient's teeth, as each tooth's landmarks are just small points encoding local geometric details. Facing this challenge, in this paper, we present an algorithm for Automatic Landmark Identification on IntraOralScans (ALIIOS) to predict 3 occlusal landmarks and 2 cervical landmarks on the upper and lower dental arches in a total of 140 landmarks, based on the segmentation of precise patch locations. In the following sections, we describe the materials, briefly review the most relevant related work, describe the study datasets, the proposed algorithm with the training and testing steps, and the results.

2 Related Work

Landmark localization remains a crucial task in both computer vision and medical imaging analysis, and the computer vision community has collectively attempted numerous approaches to address this task. Occlusion-net [7] implements an approach that encourages occlusions, where a camera can only view one side of an object (left or right, front, or back), and part of the object is outside the field of view. The framework then predicts 2D and 3D locations of occlusal key points for objects, in a largely self-supervised manner, using an off-the-shelf detector as input that is trained only on visible key point annotations. Then a graph encoder network explicitly classifies invisible edges, and a graph decoder network corrects the occluded key point locations from the initial detector. Another method uses a heatmap regression-based landmark localization on IOS datasets [10]. It incorporates the spatial configuration of anatomical landmarks at the region of interest of individual teeth to improve the robustness of the regression. Other approaches for IOS processing have determined the IOS orientation, then used the local maxima in the vertical direction for an initial approximation of the landmarks, followed by an extraction of surface gradient and curvature information to identify the shape and boundaries of each tooth. [9].

3 Method

3.1 Data

The dataset consisted of four hundred and five IOSs of the upper and lower dental arches acquired at 2 clinical centers: Universidad Corporación para Estudios en la Salud (CES) in Medellin Colombia and University of Michigan. These scans were acquired using 3Shape Trios and iTero® intraoral scanners. The scanners utilize ultrafast optical sectioning and confocal microscopy to generate 3D images from multiple 2D images with an accuracy of 6.9 ± 0.9 µm. The dataset was composed of individual anatomic shapes, patients could present one or more missing teeth and a third molar and dental appliances (braces). For each IOS, 70 maxillary dental landmarks were placed by 3 experienced clinicians on each arch, using the markups module in 3D Slicer 4.11 [6]. For each IOS, we recovered important information useful for the training steps and included the vertices, faces of the mesh, label of each face (or the positions of the landmarks), and the normal vector for each vertex.

3.2 Pre-processing

The IOSs were pre-processed using an open-source tool in 3D Slicer 4.11 [6], DentalModelSeg [4], to segment and assign the universal numbering to each tooth respectively. The scan pre-processing allowed the selection of each tooth to predict landmark placement (Fig. 1).

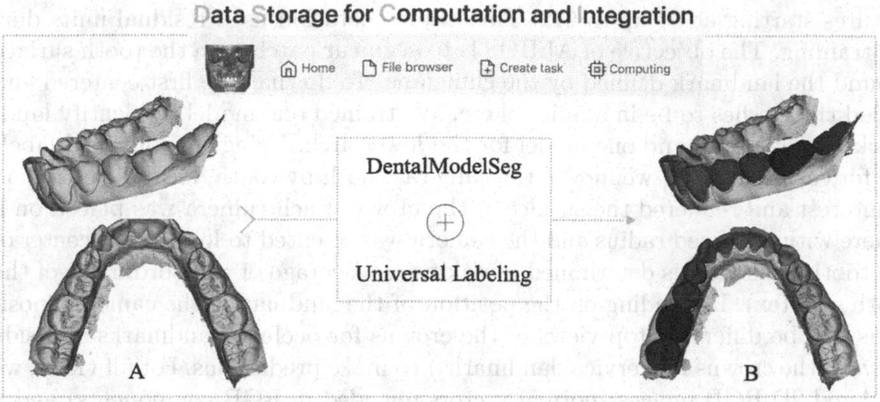

Fig. 1. IOS pre-processing A. IOS acquired using iTero® or 3Shape scanners B. Segmentation of the dental crowns with the two open-source tools: DentalModelSeg and Universal Labelling [4] to segment and assign the universal numbering.

3.3 Rendering 2D Views

We used PyTorch3D framework that allows fast 3D data representation and batching, *i.e.,* there are no intermediate pre-processing steps on the input meshes. This library was used to perform end-to-end training by rendering images of the IOS meshes that are fed to the ALIIOS convolutional neural network (CNN). PyTorch3D renderers are designed to be modular, extensible, and ready to perform gradient computation. The renderers are based on two principles:

- **Rasterizer:** The rasterization consists of projecting a 3D object on a 2D image. It uses a camera such as the FoVPerspectiveCamera which was used following the OpenGL convention for perspective and orthographic cameras. This camera is by default in the NDC coordinate system, which is a normalized coordinate system that confines in a volume the rendered part of the object/scene. In this work, we used 224×224 pixels images with a 120° FOV which allowed us to take perfect 2D views of the target area. As well as the image, the rasterizer outputs a look-up table that links each pixel on the rendered image to a corresponding face on the mesh.
- **Shaders:** The shaders are used to apply texturing/shading/blending on the rasterized images. It needs a light source as well as textures on the meshes. In this work, to generate the input images, we placed a light source in front of the 3D model, and used the normal at each vertex (encoded in RGB components) as the texture of the mesh. The mesh renderer is a Pytorch3D "HardPhong-Shading" shader.

3.4 Training

We trained a residual U-Net [8] architecture from Monai, with 4 down-sampling steps and 4 up-samplings, kernel 3×3 and stride 2, with an increasing number of features starting at 64 up to 512. This implementation used residual units during training. The objective of ALIIOS is to segment patches on the tooth surface around the landmark defined by the clinicians. To do that, we first centered and scaled the meshes to be in a unit sphere. We trained one model to identify landmarks in the upper and one model for the lower arch. Using the universal labeling for each crown, [4] we moved the cameras tooth by tooth, located the region of interest and rendered the surface of the crown. Each camera was placed on a sphere with a defined radius and the camera was oriented to look at the center of the tooth (this view is determined by taking the average of all coordinates of the tooth's vertex). Depending on the position of the landmarks, the cameras' positions will be different (top views of the crowns for occlusal landmarks and side views of the crowns for cervical landmarks) to make predictions. For all views, we rendered 2D RGB images (normal vectors encoded in RGB components) and a depth map as a fourth channel. These images are then fed to the ALIIOS U-Net (Fig. 2 A). These depth maps were grayscale representations of the distance of the faces to the cameras. For the ground truth, we used the pix-to-face lookup table to retrieve the corresponding labeled images of uniform patches with unique colors for each type of landmark (Fig. 2 B). We used DiceCEloss to compare similarities between the output and the ground truth and the ADAM optimization algorithm for stochastic gradient descent. The learning rate was 1e−4, with a batch size of ten for the occlusal landmarks and a batch size of one for the cervical landmarks. To train each model, 6 GB of the GPU was used and the training took an average of 5 h. The training was done on a workstation with 2 NVIDIA Corporation GP102 [TITAN Xp] graphic cards, Intel® Core™ i7-8700K CPU @ 3.70 GHz × 12 processors, and 2 TB disk capacity.

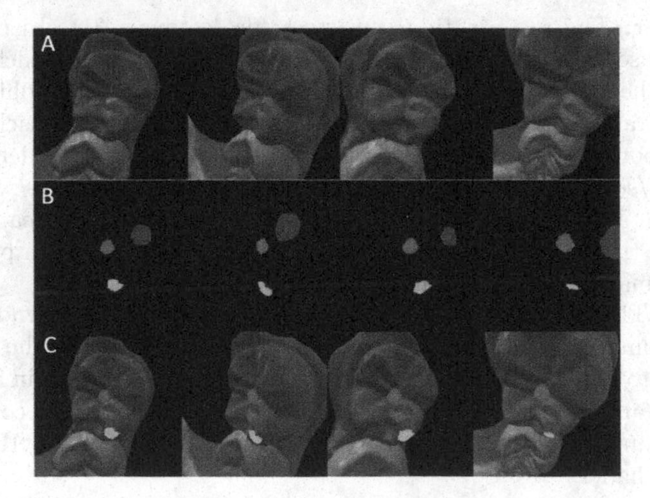

Fig. 2. A.U-Net input images. B.U-Net output patches. C.Identification of the surface meshes vertices using the U-Net output.

3.5 Prediction

To predict the landmarks on an IOS, after the segmentation with universal labeling, we moved the cameras to adequate positions. The 2D images generated by the renderer were set as input of the ALIIOS U-Net. To improve accuracy, post-processing steps were applied to the output to clean the pixels of the patches incorrectly placed on adjacent teeth. Only the faces that belong to the target tooth remained. Using the “pix to face” function on the segmented patches, we identified the faces corresponding to each pixel of the patches. For each patch color, we collected all the corresponding faces and averaged all vertices coordinates to find an approximated position. The final predicted landmark position was identified as the closest point to the approximated point on the mesh surface, saved as a fiducial list that contains all the landmarks.

4 Results

To test the performance of the ALIIOS approach in our entire dataset, we performed a 5-fold cross-validation, each time using a different 20% portion of the available data as a test set that was not included in the training. A fiducial list was generated with the predicted positions of the landmarks in about 1 min. To compute the prediction accuracy, we compared the distance between the clinicians’ landmarks and the predicted landmarks. The clinically acceptable distance range that landmark prediction should not exceed is 1 mm. Figure 3 shows the average accuracy for each tooth in the lower jaw. Table 1 summarizes the accuracy of each different model. A violin plot of each type of model is presented below in Fig. 4 to 7.

Table 1. Accuracy results table for occlusal and cervical landmarks on lower and upper arches

	Upper	Lower
Occlusal	0.45 ± 0.28 mm	0.43 ± 0.28 mm
Cervical	0.62 ± 0.28 mm	0.62 ± 0.28 mm

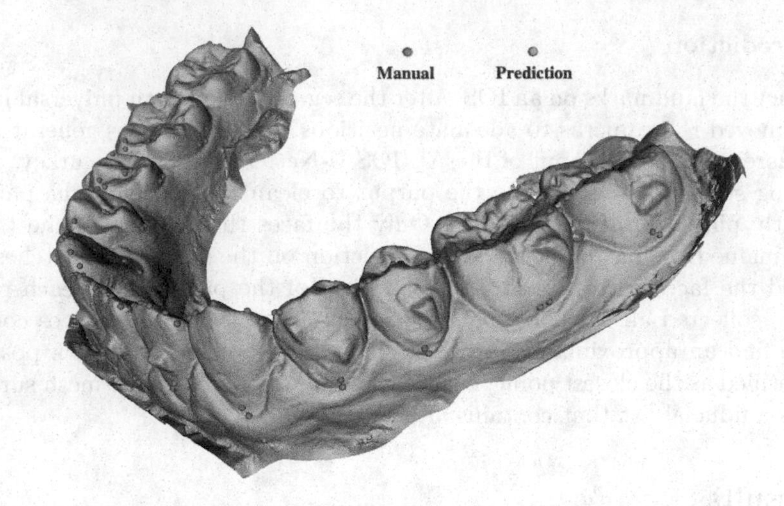

Fig. 3. Comparison between manual landmarks and predicted on the lower arch. The red spheres represent the clinician's landmarks (manual) and the green spheres are the ones predicted by ALIIOS. The diagram displays the average error (mm) for each landmark. (Color figure online)

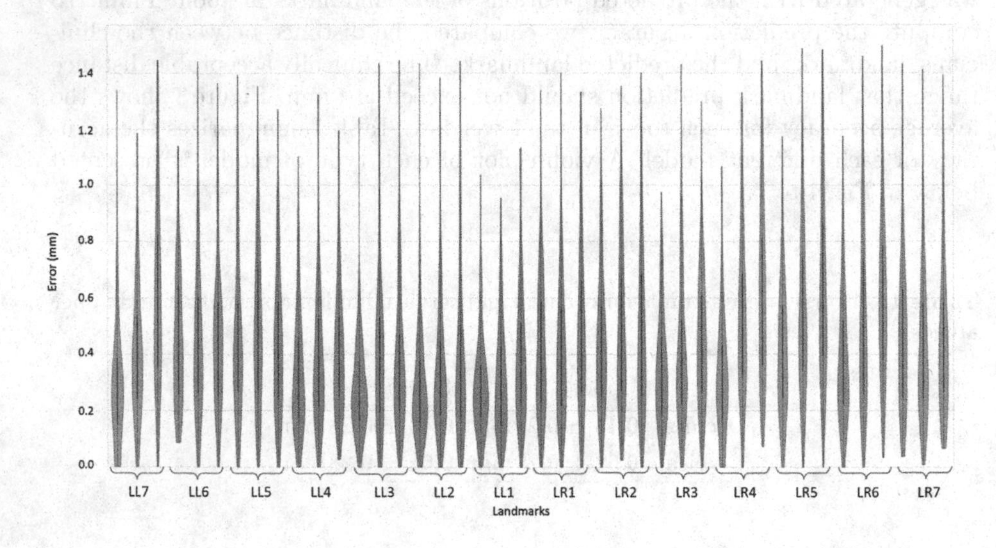

Fig. 4. Accuracy for the lower occlusal landmarks.

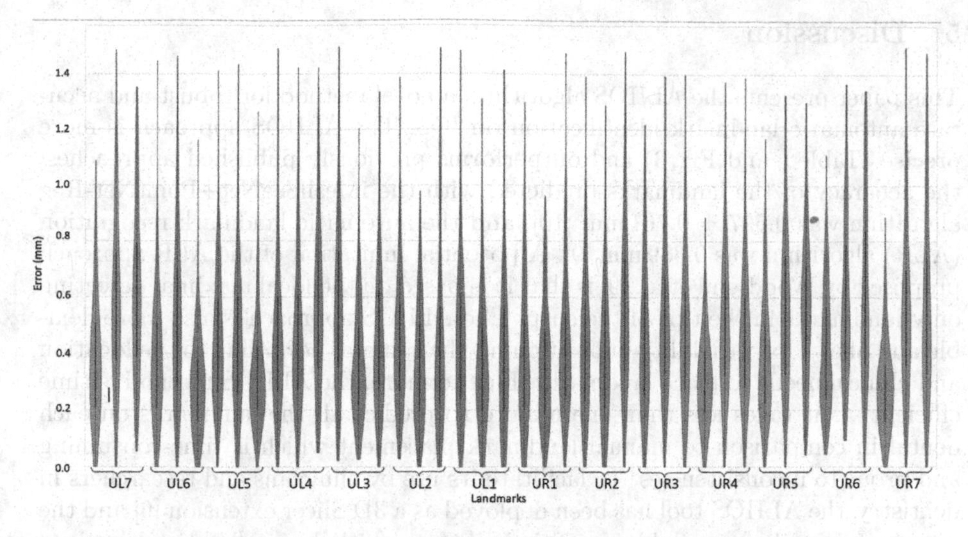

Fig. 5. Accuracy for the upper occlusal landmarks.

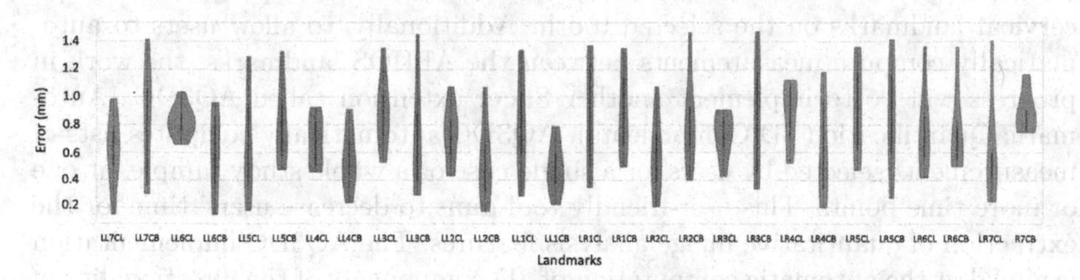

Fig. 6. Accuracy for the lower cervical landmarks.

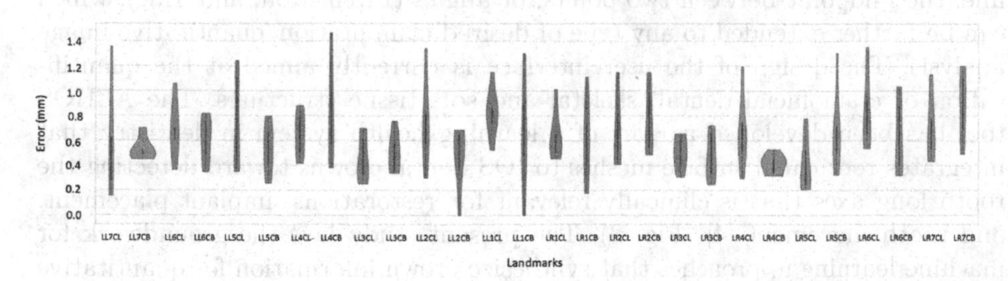

Fig. 7. Accuracy for the upper cervical landmarks.

Landmark name description: The first letter represents upper or lower. The second character represents left or right. Then the tooth number and finally the landmark type. In Fig. 4 and 5, each tooth has, from left to right, occlusal, mesial buccal, and distal buccal landmarks. In Fig. 6 and 7, "CL" stands for cervical langual and "CB" stands for cervical buccal.

5 Discussion

This paper presents the ALIIOS algorithm, a novel method for robust and accurate automatic landmark identification on IOS. The ALIIOS approach is more precise (Table 1 and Fig. 3) and outperforms previously published approaches: the accuracy of the landmarks predicted with the iMeshSegNet+PointNet-Reg algorithm was 0.597 ± 0.761 mm [10], and the automatic landmark recognition (ALR) algorithm was 0.389 mm [9]. A potential limitation of the ALR approach proposed by Woodsend et al. [9] is that it is based on the local maxima, detecting only landmarks in the tips of the cusp. The ALIIOS approach is also more flexible and allows for variability in positioning the cameras according to the location and clinical needs to place landmarks. Furthermore, the ALIIOS method is time efficient, as it takes less than one minute to predict all the landmarks on each dental in comparison to manual landmark placement which is time-consuming and prone to inconsistencies. To facilitate its use by clinicians and researchers in dentistry, the ALIIOS tool has been deployed as a 3D Slicer extension [6] and the open-source code is available on Github (https://github.com/baptistebaquero/ALIDDM.git). The ALIIOS intuitive interface allows users to predict occlusal or cervical landmarks on the selected tooth. Additionally, to allow users to automatically compute measurements between the ALIIOS landmarks, the work in progress will be to implement another Slicer extension called AQ3DC (Automatic Quantification 3D Components). AQ3DC automatically computes lists of measurements selected by users for a single case or a whole study sample, at one or more time points. This user-friendly tool aims to decrease users' time for the extraction of quantitative image analysis features. The AQ3DC implementation is aimed at the automatic computation of 3D components of the directionality of distances (Anteroposterior, Right/Left, Supeoinferior) between points, point to line, the midpoint between two points, or angles (Pitch, Roll, and Yaw), which can be further extended to any type of desired computation/quantitative image analysis. The design of the user interface is currently aimed at the quantification of craniofacial dental, skeletal and soft tissue structures. The ALIIOS tool has been developed as part of a learning health system in dentistry that integrates root canal surface meshes to IOS dental crowns toward detecting the tooth long axes that is clinically relevant for restorations, implant placement, and tooth movement [4] (Fig. 8). The present study lays the groundwork for machine learning approaches that synthesize crown information for quantitative assessments. Future studies will utilize multi-modality merging and annotation of cone-beam CT and IOS scans for challenging craniofacial applications that require both imaging modalities.

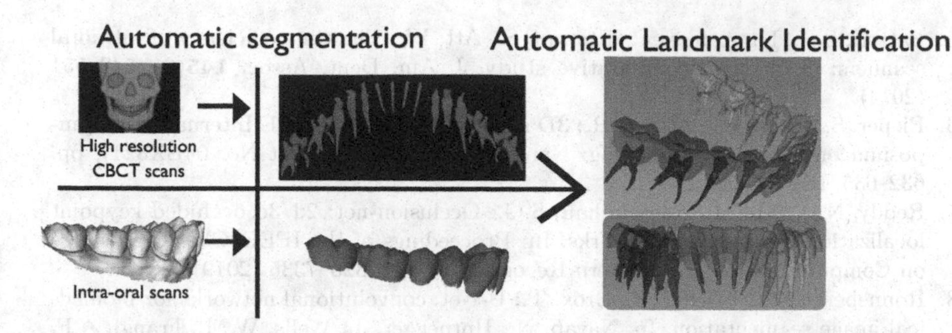

Fig. 8. Proposed future work: Segmentation of root canal and prediction of the tooth long axis.

6 Conclusion

We developed and validated a novel ALIIOS algorithm to automatically identify teeth landmarks on IOS. Our algorithm is optimized using Monai and PyTorch libraries. The ALIIOS predicts the location of landmark patches and identifies the final precise landmark position following post-processing steps. Our method has a precision of 0.43 ± 0.28 mm and 0.45 ± 0.28 mm for respectively lower and upper occlusal landmarks, and 0.62 ± 0.28 mm for lower and upper cervical landmarks. Overall, these findings demonstrate the clinical application of ALIIOS to more automated quantitative 3D imaging assessments in dental research and practice.

Acknowledgments. Supported by NIDCR R01 024450, AA0F Dewel Memorial Biomedical Research award by Research Enhancement Award Activity 141 from the University of the Pacific, Arthur A. Dugoni School of Dentistry, and the American Association of Orthodontists Foundation (AAOF).

References

1. Burhardt, L., Livas, C., Kerdijk, W., van der Meer, W.J., Ren, Y.: Treatment comfort, time perception, and preference for conventional and digital impression techniques: a comparative study in young patients. Am. J. Orthod. Dentofac. Orthop. **150**(2), 261–267 (2016)
2. Chiu, A., Chen, Y.W., Hayashi, J., Sadr, A.: Accuracy of cad/cam digital impressions with different intraoral scanner parameters. Sensors **20**(4), 1157 (2020)
3. Cong, A., et al.: Dental long axes using digital dental models compared to cone-beam computed tomography. Orthod. Craniofac. Res. **25**(1), 64–72 (2022)
4. Deleat-Besson, R., et al.: Automatic segmentation of dental root canal and merging with crown shape. In: 2021 43rd Annual International Conference of the IEEE Engineering in Medicine & Biology Society (EMBC), pp. 2948–2951. IEEE (2021)

5. Patzelt, S.B., Lamprinos, C., Stampf, S., Att, W.: The time efficiency of intraoral scanners: an in vitro comparative study. J. Am. Dent. Assoc. **145**(6), 542–551 (2014)
6. Pieper, S., Halle, M., Kikinis, R.: 3D slicer. In: 2004 2nd IEEE International Symposium on Biomedical Imaging: Nano to Macro (IEEE Cat No. 04EX821), pp. 632–635. IEEE (2004)
7. Reddy, N.D., Vo, M., Narasimhan, S.G.: Occlusion-net: 2d/3d occluded keypoint localization using graph networks. In: Proceedings of the IEEE/CVF Conference on Computer Vision and Pattern Recognition, pp. 7326–7335 (2019)
8. Ronneberger, O., Fischer, P., Brox, T.: U-Net: convolutional networks for biomedical image segmentation. In: Navab, N., Hornegger, J., Wells, W.M., Frangi, A.F. (eds.) MICCAI 2015. LNCS, vol. 9351, pp. 234–241. Springer, Cham (2015). https://doi.org/10.1007/978-3-319-24574-4_28
9. Woodsend, B., et al.: Development of intra-oral automated landmark recognition (ALR) for dental and occlusal outcome measurements. European J. Orthod. **44**(1), 43–50 (2022)
10. Wu, T.H., et al.: Two-stage mesh deep learning for automated tooth segmentation and landmark localization on 3D intraoral scans. arXiv preprint arXiv:2109.11941 (2021)
11. Zimmermann, M., Ender, A., Mehl, A.: Local accuracy of actual intraoral scanning systems for single-tooth preparations in vitro. J. Am. Dent. Assoc. **151**(2), 127–135 (2020)

STAU-Net: A Spatial Structure Attention Network for 3D Coronary Artery Segmentation

Guanjie Tong[1], Haijun Lei[1], Limin Huang[1], Zhihui Tian[1], Hai Xie[2], Baiying Lei[2(✉)], and Longjiang Zhang[3(✉)]

[1] Guangdong Province Key Laboratory of Popular High Performance Computers, College of Computer Science and Software Engineering, Shenzhen University, Shenzhen 518060, China

[2] National- Regional Key Technology Engineering Laboratory for Medical Ultrasound, Guangdong Key Laboratory for Biomedical Measurements and Ultrasound Imaging, School of Biomedical Engineering, Health Science Center, Shenzhen University, Shenzhen 518060, China

leiby@szu.edu.cn

[3] Department of Radiology, Jinling Hospital, Medical School of Nanjing University, Nanjing 210002, Jiangsu, China

kevinzhlj@163.com

Abstract. Automated segmentation of coronary artery is critical yet challenging for the detection and quantification of cardiovascular diseases. Considering the limitation of computing power, most existing 3D coronary artery segmentation methods divide original data into patches or 2D slices for segmentation to support the limited GPU memory, thereby causing limited segmentation performance due to the loss of contextual information of coronary artery structure. To solve above issues, this paper proposes a novel model for 3D coronary artery segmentation by enhancing structural information of features. Specifically, the proposed framework consists of a structure attention fusion (STAF) block and up-sample fusion (UF) block. The STAF block utilizes channel attention and spatial attention to enhance the fused feature maps from the output of dilated convolution at adjacent scales, and the UF block offsets the loss contextual information by fusing the feature map of the upper decoder. Also, the framework first resamples the input to a fixed size to implement training and up-sample to original size by customized post-processing at output stage. Compared with other related segmentation networks, the results demonstrate that our method can segment more detailed information of coronary artery tree and achieve better performance.

Keywords: Coronary artery segmentation · Structural attention · Feature fusion

Y. Chen et al. (Eds.): CLIP 2022, LNCS 13746, pp. 43–53, 2023.
https://doi.org/10.1007/978-3-031-23179-7_5

1 Introduction

Cardiovascular disease is one of the diseases with the highest mortality rate in the world, which has become a global medical concern in recent years [1]. The segmentation of coronary artery is essential to the medical clinical diagnosis and still a quite challenging task due to the complexity of coronary artery trees and the small size of vessels. The coronary angiography utilizes the imaging function of the angiography machine, through percutaneous puncture of the radial artery in the wrist or the femoral artery at the root of the thigh, the special angiography catheter will be retrograded to the root of the ascending aorta along the aorta, and then explore and align with the left or right coronary artery orifice, and inject the contrast agent under multiple different projection angles. Hence, the overall structure can be analyzed by rendering the coronary Computer tomography (CT) angiography for clinical auxiliary diagnosis [2]. Segmenting the 3D coronary artery wall and lumen can obtain accurate anatomical and morphological information about the plaque of vessels, especially the severity of coronary stenosis. However, the post-process needs to be carried out in a radiology workstation, and the segmentation and reconstruction of coronary artery tree are time-consuming and cumbersome. It is possible to overcome these problems by using fully automated coronary artery reconstruction and allow rapid processing of even large amounts of Coronary Computed Tomography Angiogram (CCTA) data.

It's time-consuming and cumbersome for coronary artery segmentation by using manual or semi-automatic methods due to the high resolution of CCTA images. Therefore, there is an urgent demand to develop an automatic and effective method that can accurately segment coronary artery from CCTA images. Since the inherent noise of images, the similarity between the target features and the complex background of the coronary artery make it very difficult to segment the salient object. To solve this issue, various algorithms for coronary artery segmentation have been proposed in the past decade. For example, Kerkeni et al. proposed a region growth rule by utilizing vascular extension properties and direction information in a unique way for the segmentation of vessel tree [3]. Lesage et al. presented a new Bayesian tracking algorithm based on particle filter to depict coronary artery from CT angiography [4]. Kang et al. developed and validated mathematically derived morphological criteria based myocardial segmentation using intravascular ultrasound (IVUS) parameters and affected myocardial regions [5]. Although these methods have achieved good performance, these methods are not extensible. For instance, those traditional methods are difficult to achieve good performance when the data scale is massive and characteristics of the data are not obvious.

Deep learning algorithms have been rapidly developed to solve different problems related to medical image field, such as image registration [6], image segmentation [7] and image retrieval [8,9]. Among them, the methods based on deep learning with convolutional neural network have achieved good performance in several image segmentation tasks. For example, fully convolutional networks (FCN) [10], U-Net [11] and Dense-UNet [12] are proposed to accomplish the medical image segmentation. In order to fully extract the spatial structure features of multidimensional medical data, researchers designed many segmentation models based on 3D convolutional neural network, such as 3D-FCN, 3D U-Net [13] and V-Net [14]. For coronary artery segmentation, many methods based on 3D convolution are proposed to extract structure. For example, Liang et al. proposed a new 3D semi supervised architecture, which utilizes the time information of video to segment coronary artery from angiographic video and combines the characteristics of the 3D coronary artery tree from 3D U-Net and 2D U-Net through the dimension conversion module and context extraction module. As a result, a clear and complete coronary artery structure is extracted [15]. For the CCTA data, there are the following challenges: 1) the background of the medical image information is complex, 2) the overall pixel size of CCTA data is big, 3) the coronary artery feature information is not as obvious as that of natural images. To address it, the used common methods are to divide the input image into several patches or slice the input and send them into the network. In summary, most existing frameworks divide each part of the data separately and restore the results with the original size, or divide the 3D data into several 2D slices and employ network to segment 2D slices, and finally these segmented slices are recovered to 3D segmentation maps. Although these methods meet the requirements of computational power and achieve good performance in the field of medical image segmentation, these proposed methods do not fully study the 3D structural features of coronary artery tree, which causes it is difficult to accurately segment 3D coronary artery, for the reason that the 2D methods or 3D patches lack contextual information and feature representation.

To address these issues, we propose a novel 3D coronary artery segmentation model, called STAU-Net, which attempts to make full use of the similarity of 3D coronary artery tree at different scales. The STAU-Net has powerful feature extraction ability for 3D coronary artery by employing STAF and UF blocks. Meanwhile, we design a post-processing method that using median filtering smooth resampling back to the original size prediction map and constructing the largest connected region to eliminate some false segmentation results of the model to restore the segmentation results of structure of coronary artery. The blood vessel boundary after resampling is smoothed through median filtering, and then the holes in the segmented vessels are eliminated by constructing the method of maximum connected region and image morphology, and then get the final result. Additionally, we fuse the feature maps of each stage of decoder to enhance the local and global information. Compared with other related 3D segmentation models, our approach achieves better performance.

2 Methods

In this section, we first introduce our proposed STAU-Net for 3D coronary artery segmentation. Subsequently, we describe the devised STAF block in detail.

2.1 STAU-Net

By our investigation, 3D coronary artery has similar spatial structures at different scales. The proposed method uses the similarity of the vascular tree with different scales to resample the data to a fixed size to fit the computational power. Finally, the method of image morphology is employed to construct connected domain to restore the size of output as the original size. The schematic illustration of our framework is show in Fig. 1.

The input images are resized into a fixed scale to train the model, which is then fed into the STAU-Net, STAU-Net adopts the traditional encoder-decoder structure, which is similar to the 3D U-Net [13]. The STAF block is designed to strengthen the feature extraction of coronary artery tree, and the segmentation results are restored to the original size through special post-processing without changing the overall structure. For the convolution module of the encoder, we employ 3D convolution with residual structure, instance normalization, and ReLU activation. For the decoder, each up-sample convolution block consists of a transpose convolution and instance normalization. To enhance the feature expression between the encoder and decoder, the extracted features are concatenated through STAF to enhance the feature expression.

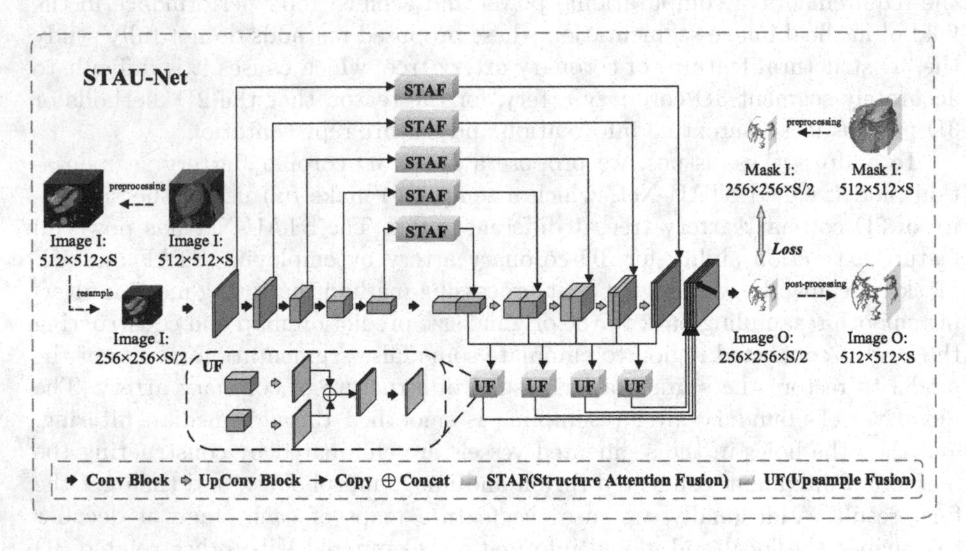

Fig. 1. Architecture of our proposed framework. The 3D CCTA data is preprocessed as the input of the framework. The STAF and UF modules are devised to strengthen feature extraction.

In order to make full use of the contextual information of spatial structure, we perform up-sample fusion (UF) operation on the feature maps of the adjacent decoding modules to strengthen the details of feature maps. Feature pyramid network (FPN) [16] is a common method for multi-scale feature fusion, which has been widely used in many fields. The structure of FPN combines the features of different levels to integrate semantic features of different scales through horizontal connection. Similar to FPN, we enhance the feature information by sampling and fusing the features of adjacent decoding modules to the output size, for the reason that the adjacent features have similar semantic information, and UF module is reused to fuse the feature maps to reduce the loss of the semantic information in the transmission by adjacent decoding modules. Finally, all the feature maps are weighted to get the segmentation result.

2.2 Structure Attention Fusion Block

In the stage of training, the spatial details are often lost in the output results with high-dimension due to cascaded convolution. The loss of spatial information makes it difficult to segment the small branches of coronary artery. Therefore, we propose a STAF block to solve this issue, which is shown in Fig. 2. The atrous convolution of different scales is employed to handle the feature maps,

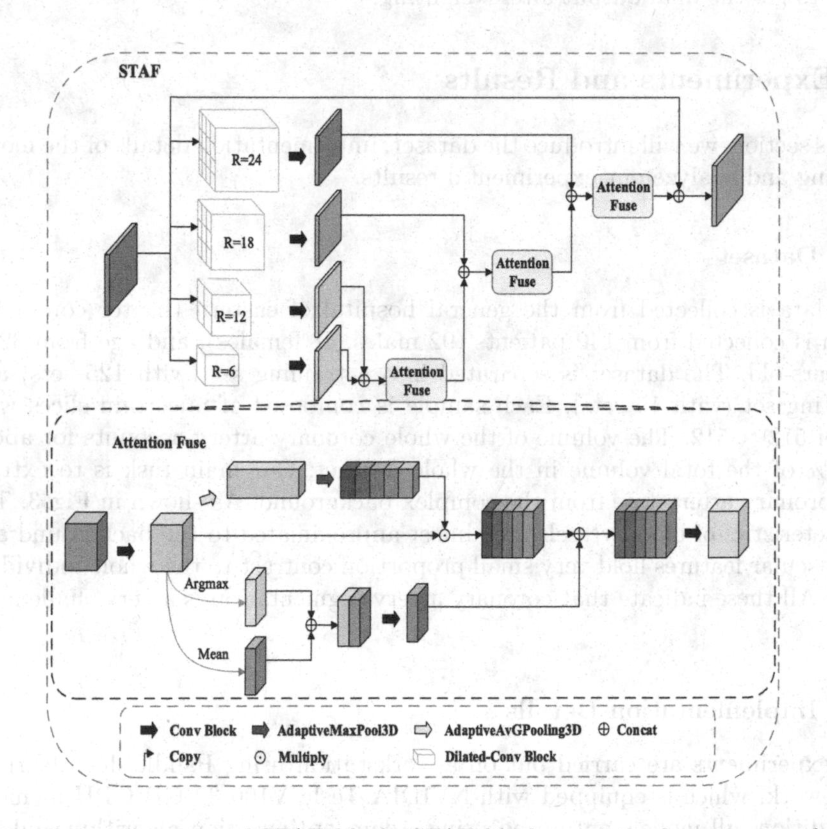

Fig. 2. The architecture of STAF block. STAF block consists of atrous convolution and attention fuse block. Attention fuse is used to enhance the feature from the adjacent atrous convolution by combining channel attention module and spatial attention module.

which is similar to atrous spatial pyramid pooling (ASPP). The extracted feature structures from the feature maps with similar scale are always relevant, which are performed by channel splicing. Subsequently, the obtained features are input to the feature fusion module, which is utilized to extract spatial and channel features by 3D channel attention and spatial attention modules. Unlike the convolutional block attention module (CBAM) [17], CBAM emphasizes the meaningful characteristics of the two main dimensions of the channel and space axis and apply channel attention and spatial attention modules to weight feature maps in turn. These two attention modules are employed in the 3D segmentation model, in which the two feature maps are weighted, respectively. Due to the complexity of 3D model spatial structure, we perform the channel attention and spatial attention to the fuse the extracted feature maps, whose advantage is that the operation can better maintain the integrity of 3D feature structure of coronary artery. In order to decrease the complexity of the module, we first use the $1 \times 1 \times 1$ convolution operation to compress the channel of input, then fuse the obtained feature maps level by level, which is multiplied by the input feature maps to get the final output after weighting.

3 Experiments and Results

In this section, we will introduce the dataset, implementation details of the model training and analyze our experimental results.

3.1 Dataset

The data is collected from the general hospital of eastern theater command, which is collected from 140 patients (92 males, 48 females), and age from 32 to 90 years-old. The dataset is separated into a training set (with 125 sets) and a testing set (with 15 sets). Each sample is composed of uncertain slices with size of 512×512. The volume of the whole coronary artery accounts for about 0.165% of the total volume in the whole dataset. Our main task is to extract the coronary artery tree from the complex background. As shown in Fig. 3. The characteristics of blood vessels are almost approximated to the background and the vascular features hold very small proportion contrast to the whole individual pixel. All these indicate that coronary artery segmentation is a very challenging task.

3.2 Implementation Details

The experiments are carried out on a workstation using Paddle deep learning framework, which is equipped with NVIDIA Tesla V100 32 GB GPU memory. In addition, all models optimized using Adam optimization algorithm and the initial learning rate is 0.0005. The procedure of whole training takes 20 h for 200 epochs. For the pre-processing of dataset, we first convert the format Digital Imaging and Communications in Medicine (DICOM) to the format NIFTI by using SimpleITK and resize it to a fixed size. We adjust the heat unit (HU) value to 0–1000 as the input after normalization. In the post-processing stage, we use median filtering to smooth resampling back to the original size prediction map and construct the largest connected region to eliminate some false segmentation results of the model. In addition, we also use image morphology to fill the holes in the segmented blood vessels. In the stage of training, the cross entropy and soft dice losses are combined by same weight, in which L_{ce} donates entropy loss function and L_{s_dice} donates soft dice loss function. The total loss function is defined as:

$$L_{loss} = L_{ce} + L_{s\_dice}, \tag{1}$$

The L_{ce} is defined as follows:

$$L_{ce} = -\frac{1}{whd}\sum_{k=0}^{d-1}\sum_{j=0}^{w-1}\sum_{i=0}^{h-1} p(k,i,j)log(\hat{p}(k,i,j)), \tag{2}$$

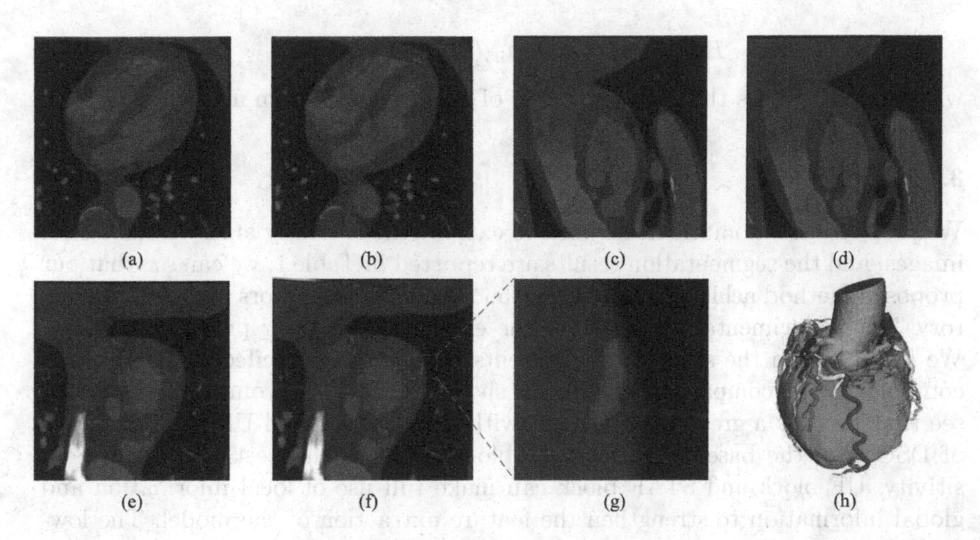

Fig. 3. A sample that slices from different views with the corresponding ground truth and the overall structure of the heart. (a), (c), (e) represent slices from different views and (b), (d), (f) are the overlap of the original image and the corresponding ground truth, respectively. (h) shows the complex heart structure in the computed tomography angiogram diagram.

where d, w, h are the dimensions of each input, $p(k,i,j)$ indicates the input 3D scan and $\hat{p}(k,i,j)$ denotes the output prediction at a specific pixel location (k,i,j). The soft dice loss function is defined as:

$$L_{s\_dice} = 1 - \frac{2x|D_{pre} \cap D_{gt}| + \epsilon}{|D_{pre}| + |D_{gt}| + \epsilon}, \tag{3}$$

3.3 Evaluation Metrics

In this paper, the main evaluation metrics consist of the dice score coefficient (DSC) and the 95th-percentile of the Hausdorff distance (HD). DSC is sensitive to the internal filling of mask, while HD is sensitive to the segmented boundary. The DSC is a measure of the spatial overlap between the segmentation result S and the ground truth G, which is defined by

$$DSC(G,S) = \frac{2|G \cap S|}{|G| + |S|}, \tag{4}$$

where S is the prediction map; G is the ground truth. DSC index indicates the similarity between the segmentation result and ground truth, and the DSC value is positively correlated with the segmentation quality. The HD measures the maximal distance between the segmentation results and the ground truth, the HD is negatively correlated with segmentation performance. To improve the robustness of the conventional HD, we use the 95th percentile of the distances to suppress the outliers, and HD is expressed as

$$HD(G,S) = max h_{95}(G,S), h_{95}(S,G), \tag{5}$$

where $h_{95}(G,S)$, is the 95th percentile of the distances from all $s \epsilon S$ to G .

3.4 Result

We propose an automatic framework to extract the coronary artery from CCTA images, and the segmentation results are reported in Table 1, we can see that our proposed method achieves a DSC of 80.56 and other indicators are also satisfactory. The experimental results show the effectiveness of our proposed method. We also perform the ablation experiments to evaluate the effectiveness of each component, the comparison results are shown in Table 2. From Table 2, we can see that there is a great improvement with STAF block and UF block in terms of DSC, and the baseline with STAF block achieves the best HD95 and Sensitivity. UF block and STAF block can make full use of local information and global information to strengthen the feature extraction of the model. The low-level semantic information in the encoder and decoder is enhanced by STAF block and UF block, respectively. We can see that although each component can improve HD95, the HD95 indicator of the overall framework is not significantly improved compared with other model in the ablation experiments. For the reason that the use of the two components increases the complexity of the model, resulting in much attention being paid to the interior of the vascular branches. In addition, we compare the convergence of our proposed model with other segmentation models, which is shown in Fig. 4. We can see that our model is easier to converge and the whole training process is relatively stable.

In order to further verify the effectiveness of our model, we also visualize the results of our method compared to other models on three typical examples, which are shown in Fig. 5, we can observe that the proposed method can segment

Table 1. The comparison performance of STAU-Net and other related models (%).

Method	DSC	HD95 (mm)	Sen	Jaccard	Pre	Spec
U-Net	79.10	**5.49**	78.65	65.58	79.62	99.96
Res-Unet	79.27	5.55	78.47	65.80	80.18	99.96
Dense-Unet	72.71	9.49	68.87	57.38	77.42	99.96
Vnet	78.63	5.55	**80.97**	64.92	76.55	99.96
Segnet	60.26	9.34	49.11	43.14	68.92	99.95
Ours	**80.56**	6.07	79.28	**67.07**	**81.05**	**99.97**

Table 2. The segmentation performance of ablation experiments of the used modules (%).

Baseline	STAF	UF	DSC	HD95 (mm)	Sen	Jaccard	Pre	Spec
✓			79.10	5.49	78.65	65.58	79.62	99.96
✓	✓		79.92	5.47	**81.76**	65.80	78.21	99.96
✓		✓	79.27	**5.26**	79.21	65.80	79.43	99.96
✓	✓	✓	**80.56**	6.07	79.28	**67.07**	**81.05**	**99.97**

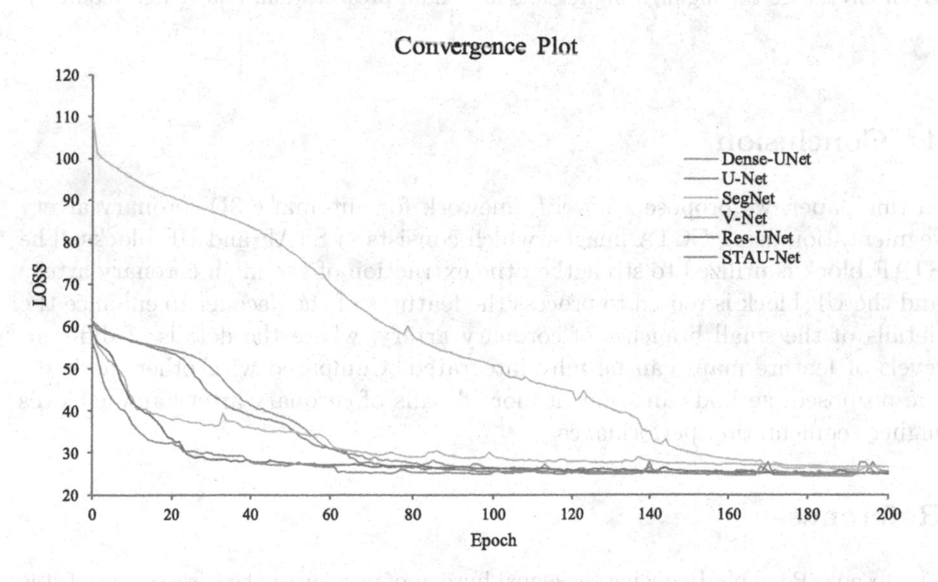

Fig. 4. The convergence of the comparative methods: SegNet, Dense-UNet, U-Net, V-Net, Res-UNet, STAU-Net. The convergence of STAU-Net is faster compared to all other methods.

more small branches of coronary artery compared with other methods from the highlighting regions with green circles. In the last column of Fig. 5, the overlap is the visual predicted results overlaps with the ground truth, the red region and the green region respectively represent the predicted results and ground truth, the overlap also shows the accuracy of our method.

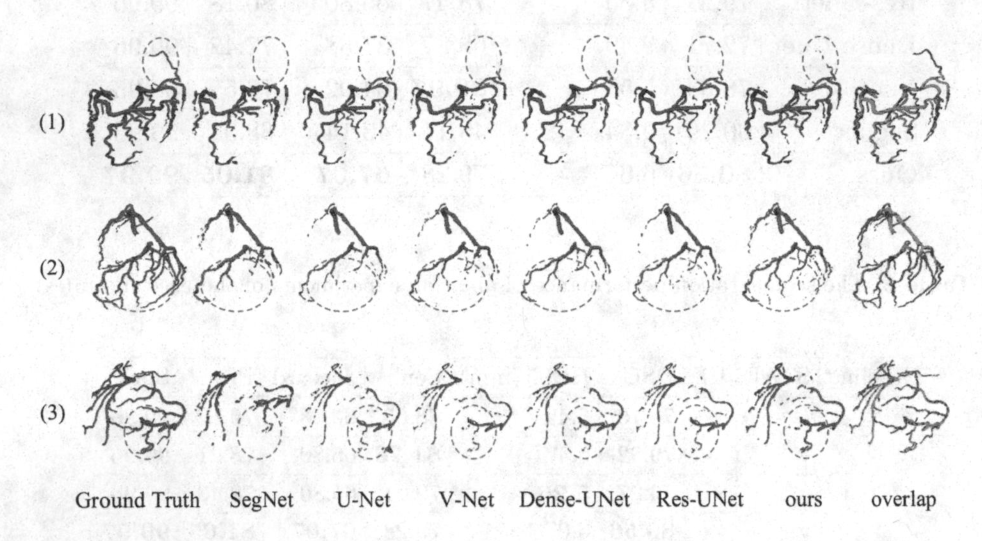

Fig. 5. The comparison results of three typical subjects by different methods. The green circles are the highlighting regions for visual presentation. (Color figure online)

4 Conclusion

In this paper, we propose a novel framework for automatic 3D coronary artery segmentation using CCTA images, which consists of STAF and UF blocks. The STAF block is utilized to strengthen the extraction of the main coronary artery and the UF block is reused to process the features of the decoder to enhance the details of the small branches of coronary artery, where the details of different levels of feature maps can be fully integrated. Compared with other methods, the proposed method can segment more details of coronary artery and achieves higher segmentation performance.

References

1. Joseph, P., et al.: Reducing the global burden of cardiovascular disease, part 1: the epidemiology and risk factors. Circ. Res. **121**(6), 677–694 (2017)
2. Goo, H.W., et al.: CT of congenital heart disease: normal anatomy and typical pathologic conditions. Radiographics **23**(suppl_1), S147–S165 (2003)

3. Kerkeni, A., Benabdallah, A., Manzanera, A., Bedoui, M.H.: A coronary artery segmentation method based on multiscale analysis and region growing. Comput. Med. Imaging Graph. **48**, 49–61 (2016)
4. Lesage, D., Angelini, E.D., Funka-Lea, G., Bloch, I.: Adaptive particle filtering for coronary artery segmentation from 3D CT angiograms. Comput. Vision Image Underst. **151**, 29–46 (2016)
5. Nishi, T., et al.: Deep learning-based intravascular ultrasound segmentation for the assessment of coronary artery disease. Int. J. Cardiol. **333**, 55–59 (2021)
6. Haskins, G., Kruger, U., Yan, P.: Deep learning in medical image registration: a survey. Mach. Vision Appl. **31**(1), 1–18 (2020)
7. Chen, H., Dou, Q., Yu, L., Qin, J., Heng, P.-A.: VoxResNet: deep voxelwise residual networks for brain segmentation from 3D MR images. Neuroimage **170**, 446–455 (2018)
8. Öztürk, Ş: Class-driven content-based medical image retrieval using hash codes of deep features. Biomed. Signal Process. **68**, 102601 (2021)
9. Öztürk, Ş: Stacked auto-encoder based tagging with deep features for content-based medical image retrieval. Expert Syst. Appl. **161**, 113693 (2020)
10. Long, J., Shelhamer, E., Darrell, T.: Fully convolutional networks for semantic segmentation. In: Proceedings of the IEEE Conference on Computer Vision and Pattern Recognition. CVPR 2015, pp. 3431–3440. IEEE, Boston (2015)
11. Ronneberger, O., Fischer, P., Brox, T.: U-Net: convolutional networks for biomedical image segmentation. In: Navab, N., Hornegger, J., Wells, W.M., Frangi, A.F. (eds.) MICCAI 2015. LNCS, vol. 9351, pp. 234–241. Springer, Cham (2015). https://doi.org/10.1007/978-3-319-24574-4_28
12. Li, X., Chen, H., Qi, X., Dou, Q., Fu, C.W., Heng, P.A.: H-DenseUNet: hybrid densely connected UNet for liver and tumor segmentation from CT volumes. Trans. Med. Imaging **37**(12), 2663–2674 (2018)
13. Çiçek, Ö., Abdulkadir, A., Lienkamp, S.S., Brox, T., Ronneberger, O.: 3D U-Net: learning dense volumetric segmentation from sparse annotation. In: Ourselin, S., Joskowicz, L., Sabuncu, M.R., Unal, G., Wells, W. (eds.) MICCAI 2016. LNCS, vol. 9901, pp. 424–432. Springer, Cham (2016). https://doi.org/10.1007/978-3-319-46723-8_49
14. Milletari, F., Navab, N., Ahmadi, S.A.: V-net: fully convolutional neural networks for volumetric medical image segmentation. In: 2016 Fourth International Conference on 3D Vision. 3DV 2016, pp 565–571. IEEE, California (2016)
15. Liang, D., et al.: Semi 3D-TENet: semi 3D network based on temporal information extraction for coronary artery segmentation from angiography video. Biomed. Signal Process. Control **69**, 102894 (2021)
16. Lin, T.Y., Dollár, P., Girshick, R., He, K., Hariharan, B., Belongie, S.: Feature pyramid networks for object detection. In: Proceedings of the IEEE Conference on Computer Vision and Pattern Recognition. CVPR 2017, pp. 2117–2125. IEEE, HI (2017)
17. Woo, S., Park, J., Lee, J.-Y., Kweon, I.S.: CBAM: convolutional block attention module. In: Ferrari, V., Hebert, M., Sminchisescu, C., Weiss, Y. (eds.) ECCV 2018. LNCS, vol. 11211, pp. 3–19. Springer, Cham (2018). https://doi.org/10.1007/978-3-030-01234-2_1

Convolutional Redistribution Network for Multi-view Medical Image Diagnosis

Yuan Zhou[1], Xiaodong Yue[1,2](✉), Yufei Chen[3], Chao Ma[3,4], and Ke Jiang[1]

[1] School of Computer Engineering and Science, Shanghai University, Shanghai 200444, China
yswantfly@shu.edu.cn

[2] Artificial Intelligence Institute of Shanghai University, Shanghai University, Shanghai 200444, China

[3] College of Electronics and Information Engineering, Tongji University, Shanghai 200092, China

[4] Department of Radiology, Changhai Hospital of Shanghai, Naval Medical University, Shanghai 200433, China

Abstract. Medical data such as Computed Tomography (CT), X-ray, and Magnetic Resonance Imaging (MRI) are integral elements of medical diagnosis. Deep learning has become common in computer-aided diagnosis, however, most of these models use only single-modal data as input and cannot take full advantage of data from different modalities for diagnosis. In addition, most of the existing multi-view models only fuse the results on a single view, without fully exploring the relationships between multi-view data. To better explore the correlation between data from different modalities, we propose a generic multi-view classification model for computer-aided diagnosis on multi-view medical images. With attention mechanism, the proposed model automatically extracts essential information from multi-view data to generate a series of "good and diverse" pseudo views for integration. The experiment results show that proposed model achieves good performance on pancreatic tumor classification task as well as the OrganMNIST3D classification task of the MedMNIST public datasets.

Keywords: Multi-view learning · Convolutional neural network · Image classification

1 Introduction

There are many examples of multi-view data in medical imaging, such as data of different modalities (X-ray, CT, MRI) or data of the same modality but different phases (T1-MRI, T2-MRI, FLAIR-MRI, etc.) or data of different orthogonal views (Axial, Coronal, Sagittal of CT, etc.). How to make full use of these multi-view data to help computer-aided diagnosis based on existing deep learning models is the focus of this paper. Most of the existing deep learning models only

Y. Chen et al. (Eds.): CLIP 2022, LNCS 13746, pp. 54–61, 2023.
https://doi.org/10.1007/978-3-031-23179-7_6

support single input-output, which cannot fully utilize multi-view data. What's more, the existing multi-view models simply fuse the results obtained from each view, without fully exploiting the relationship between multi-view data in the feature extraction stage. Based on this, we propose the Convolutional Redistribution Network, the proposed model uses attention mechanism to automatically extract information from the original multi-view data. In addition, to obtain fine ensemble results, we optimize the model by consistency loss and diversity loss, so that the model can generate a series of "good and diverse" pseudo views. "Good" means that the generated features are distinguished in the respective pseudo views, and "diverse" means that the generated features should be as different as possible from other pseudo views. Finally, we apply the model to real-world medical image datasets and show that the proposed model achieves good classification performance on both 3-phase medical datasets and 3D medical datasets.

The rest of the paper is organized as follows: Sect. 2 reviews some work that applies multi-view classification models to computer-aided diagnosis. In Sect. 3, the proposed Convolutional Redistribution Network and its loss function are described. In Sect. 4 experiments on pancreatic tumor classification and Organ-MNIST3D [2,11] classification tasks are demonstrated. Section 5 concludes this paper.

2 Related Work

Sun et al. proposed a multi-view matrix decomposition approach integrating clinical features with genetic markers [7], aimed at identifying concurrently disease subtypes and their genetic associations. For Alzheimer's Disease (AD) diagnosis with Magnetic Resonance Imaging (MRI) data, Zhu et al. maps HOG features onto the space of ROI features and inputs both mapped HOG features and original ROI features to the support vector machine for AD diagnosis [17]. Setio et al. raised a novel Computer-Aided Detection (CAD) system for pulmonary nodules by using multi-view convolutional networks (ConvNets) [6], for which discriminative features were automatically learned from the training data. Bekker et al. proposed a multi-view-classifier [1], which was a two-step classification implemented by a logistic regression classifier, and then combined the two view-level indications stochastically into a single benign or malignant decision aimed at classifying clusters of breast microcalcifications as benign and malignant. Zhang et al. proposed a Multi-Layer Multi-View Classification (ML-MVC) [15] approach that treats multi-view inputs as the first layer and constructs a potential representation to explore the complex association between features and class labels for AD diagnosis. Sun et al. proposed a novel multi-view convolutional neural network (CNN) [8] that extracts ed discriminative features and effectively incorporated these features for mammographic images to improve the mammographic image classification performance. Li et al. presented a radiomics method [5] based on dilated and attention-guided residual learning for the mammographic density classification task and designed a multi-stream network architecture specifically targeting analyzing the multi-view mammograms. Zhou et al. proposed a collective deep region-based feature representation for multi-view disease diagnosis [16]. There are three innovations in this article: automated end-to-end medical biometrics system, deep region-based feature representation, and multi-view multi-disease medical biometrics diagnosis. Xu et al. proposed a deep evidential fusion method to best exploit the belief assignment and uncertainty estimation by improving the objective function and introducing an approximation of the base rate distributions [10]. This method was applied to a real-world medical image analysis task with a dataset of enhanced three-phase CT images of patients with five subtypes of pancreatic tumors.

3 Method

3.1 The Workflow of Convolutional Redistribute Network

The structure and workflow of the proposed model is shown in Fig. 1. First, the image data of each view are extracted by backbone CNN network with the supervision of cross-entropy loss to extract the features on each view separately. The features of each view are concatenated to obtain a multi-view feature representation. After that, the multi-view feature is input into Integration Network to reduce dimension and obtain a refine multi-view feature. A series of attention networks are then used to automatically extract features from the refine multi-view feature to generate pseudo views under the supervision of consistency loss and diversity loss. Finally, to facilitate optimization and classification, a uni-space network is applied to map all pseudo views to a common space.

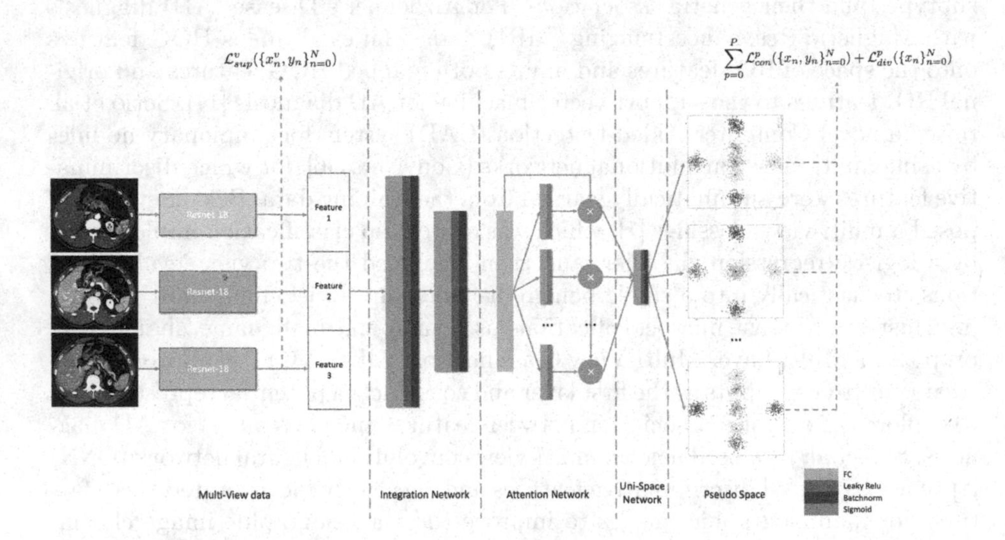

Fig. 1. The structure and workflow of Convolutional Redistribution Network.

3.2 Convolutional Redistribute Network

The multi-view data are represented as $X = \{X^{(0)}, \cdots, X^{(V)}\}$ where $X^{(V)} \in \mathbb{R}^{s^2}$ denotes the image of Vth view, s^2 denotes the image size. $Y = \{y_0, \cdots, y_n\}$ is the set of labels of all samples. The goal is to obtain a series of "good and diverse" pseudo views $\hat{Z} = \{\hat{Z^{(0)}}, \cdots, \hat{Z^{(P)}}\}$, where $\hat{Z^{(P)}} \in \mathbb{R}^{d_p \times N}$, d_p denotes the dimension of pseudo views. For a single sample, its multi-view feature is represented as concatenation after Convolutional backbone network features on all views, where d_v denotes the dimension of CNN's output:

$$x_n = [CNN(x_n^{(0)}), \cdots, CNN(x_n^{(V)})], x_n \in \mathbb{R}^{\sum_{v=0}^{V} d_v} \tag{1}$$

Refine feature representation of origin input is denoted as $\hat{x_n} = F(x_n), \hat{x_n} \in \mathbb{R}^{d_{intermediate}}$ after processed by integration network $F(x, \theta_f)$. Then, every attention network $A_p(x_i; \theta_a^p)$ gives a mask ranged $[0, 1]$ for generating pseudo view in a way of hadamard product with $\hat{x_i}$.

$$z_n^p = F(x_n) \circ A_p(x_n), z_i^p \in \mathbb{R}^{d_{intermediate}} \tag{2}$$

To use a universal metric for optimizing and classification, a uni-space network is applied to map all pseudo views to a common space $\mathbb{R}^{d_p}$. Finally, pseudo views are represented as:

$$\hat{z_n^p} = G(F(x_n) \circ A_p(x_n)), \hat{z_n^p} \in \mathbb{R}^{d_p} \tag{3}$$

After all, for a single sample X_n, the proposed model will generate P pseudo view representations $\{\hat{z_n^{(0)}}, \cdots, \hat{z_n^{(P)}}\}$.

3.3 Loss Function

To have consistent and diverse representations on each pseudo view, the loss function of the proposed model consists of three parts: $\mathcal{L}_{sup}^v$, $\mathcal{L}_{con}^p$ and $\mathcal{L}_{div}^p$. The overall loss function is formalized as:

$$\mathcal{L} = \sum_{v=0}^{V} \mathcal{L}_{sup}^v(\{x_n^v, y_n\}_{n=0}^N) + \sum_{p=0}^{P} \mathcal{L}_{con}^p(\{x_n, y_n\}_{n=0}^N) + \mathcal{L}_{div}^p(\{x_n\}_{n=0}^N) \tag{4}$$

where v denotes the vth view of input and p denotes the pth pseudo view respectively. $\{x_n\}_{n=0}^N$ denotes all sample set, $\{x_n, y_n\}_{n=0}^N$ denotes the set of sample and its label and $\{x_n^v, y_n\}_{n=0}^N$ denotes the sample set on vth view.

$\mathcal{L}_{sup}^v(\cdot)$term enables the backbone network to extract good features from multi-view image inputs for subsequent feature redistribution. Logits of vth input x_n^v retrieved from fully-connected layer can be represented as $\hat{y_n^v} = fc(CNN(x_n^v))$.

$$\mathcal{L}_{sup}^v(\{x_n^v, y_n\}_{n=0}^N) = \sum_{n=0}^{N} y_n log \hat{y_n^v} + (1 - y_n) log(1 - \hat{y_n^v}) \tag{5}$$

$\mathcal{L}_{consistency}(\cdot)$ term utilizes a euclidean distance-based contrastive learning loss to enforce features of the same class close and keep features of different classes away (at least $d_{consistency}$). Term y_{ij} is an indicator function, when i and j are same class y_{ij} is 1, else 0.

$$\begin{aligned}\mathcal{L}_{consistency}(\{x_n^p, y_n\}_{n=0}^N) = \frac{1}{N}\sum_{0\leq i<j\leq N}^{N} & (y_{ij}dis(\hat{z_i^p}, \hat{z_j^p})^2) \\ +(1-y_{ij})max(0, d_{consistency} & - dis(\hat{z_i^p}, \hat{z_j^p})^2)\end{aligned} \tag{6}$$

$\mathcal{L}_{diversity}(\cdot)$ term enforces features of different pseudo views to be as diverse as possible, where $\circ$ indicates Hadamard product. $||\cdot||_1$ denotes the sum of the absolute value of the result. If the feature representations of a sample in different pseudo views are similar, the product of this terms will be large, and vice versa it will be small. In this case, the diversity of features in different pseudo views can be guaranteed numerically.

$$\mathcal{L}_{diversity}(\{x_n\}_{n=0}^N) = \frac{1}{N}\sum_{n=0}^{N}\sum_{0\leq s<t\leq P}^{P} ||\hat{z_n^s} \circ \hat{z_n^t}||_1 \tag{7}$$

4 Experiment

4.1 Experiment on Pancreatic Tumor Classification

We applied proposed method to a real-world medical image analysis task on a dataset of enhanced 3-phase Computed Tomography (CT) images of 3 subtypes of pancreatic tumor patients collected by Changhai Hospital. The dataset consists of 50 patients with pancreatic ductal adenocarcinoma (PDAC), 50 patients with intraductal papillary mucinous neoplasm (IPMN) and 26 patients with pancreatic neuroendocrine tumor (NET), and 126 patients in total. The CT scan was performed in arterial phase (AP), venous phase (VP), and delayed phase (DP). We selected the maximum cross-section of the tumor as the region of interest for network input.

A standard ResNet18 [4] is adopted as the proposed model's backbone network and K-nearest neighbors as classifiers for each pseudo view. We use SGD with $1e^{-3}$ learning rate, 0.9 momentum and $1e^{-5}$ weight decay as optimizer. The proposed model's parameters setting is as follows: $P = 4$, $K = 5$, $d_v = 512$, $d_{intermediate} = 512$, $d_p = 256$. In this work, all method is implemented by PyTorch on one NVIDIA Geforce GTX 3090 with 24GB GPU memory.

We compare the results of ResNet18 [4] network and VIT [9] network on each phase and result of a multi-view model TMC [3]. All results are obtained by 5-fold-cross-validation. Table 1 shows the results on commonly used classification metrics. VIT-AP, VIT-DP, VIT-VP represent the performance of the VIT model on a single view of AP, DP, and VP respectively, as well as Res-AP, Res-DP, and Res-VP.

Table 1. Comparative experimental results on pancreatic tumor classification. The best results are **bolded** and the second best results are underlined

Method	Accuracy	Precision	Recall	F1-Score
VIT-AP	70.77	73.69	71.56	69.83
VIT-DP	62.31	59.34	60.67	59.11
VIT-VP	61.54	67.07	60.00	59.73
Res-AP	64.62	74.42	61.33	62.33
Res-DP	68.46	70.66	65.56	66.34
Res-VP	60.77	56.10	56.22	54.61
TMC	68.46	68.09	63.78	63.02
Proposed	**77.69**	**79.57**	**76.67**	**76.41**

4.2 Experiment on Standard Datasets

To further validate the effectiveness of the proposed model, we conduct experiments on a public dataset, OrganMNIST3D, subdataset of MedMNIST [13,14], which contains a total of 11 categories of body organs, with 972 cases in the training set and 610 cases in the test set.

To get a close result as reported in [14], we use Adam optimizer with learning rates of $1e^{-3}$, and $1e^{-5}$ weight decay in this experiment. Both the proposed and the comparison models' CNN backbone use standard ResNet18 [4]. The remaining hyperparameters and model's classifier are set as same as before.

We use three different orthogonal views (Axial, Coronal, Sagittal) as the multi-view input of the proposed model. The results of the 2D model ResNet18 on each view and the results of the 3D model ResNet18-3d [12] and the multi-view model TMC are compared, respectively. Table 2 shows the results on commonly used classification metrics. All results are obtained by averaging five random experiments. Res-A, Res-C, and Res-S represent the single-view performance of the Resnet18 model on three orthogonal views, respectively.

Table 2. Comparative experimental results on OrganMNIST3D 11 categories classification task. The best results are **bolded** and the second best results are underlined

Method	Accuracy	Precision	Recall	F1-Score
Res-A	83.80	86.61	84.94	85.52
Res-C	83.64	86.77	85.27	85.74
Res-S	67.67	71.41	70.48	70.35
Res-3d	90.72	92.32	91.38	91.69
TMC	91.05	92.91	92.42	92.56
Proposed	**93.18**	**94.41**	**93.43**	**93.76**

5 Conclusion

In this work, we proposed a generic multi-view classification model for medical image diagnosis. The proposed model use attention mechanism to fully exploit the relationships between multi-view data. With consistency and diversity loss function, model generates a series of "good and diverse" pseudo views for ensemble. The experiment results show that the proposed model has good performance on common multi-view medical cases such as 3-phase medical datasets and 3D medical datasets. Since our model does not impose restrictions on the number and modality of input views, it is possible to explore the model's performance on multi-view medical images with different modalities (X-ray, CT, MRI) or other non-medical multi-view images in the future as well.

Acknowledgements. This work was supported by National Natural Science Foundation of China (Serial Nos. 61976134, 62173252), Natural Science Foundation of Shanghai (NO.21ZR1423900) and Open Project Foundation of Intelligent Information Processing Key Laboratory of Shanxi Province, China (No. CICIP2021001).

References

1. Bekker, A.J., Shalhon, M., Greenspan, H., Goldberger, J.: Multi-view probabilistic classification of breast microcalcifications. IEEE Trans. Med. Imaging **35**(2), 645–653 (2015)
2. Bilic, P., Christ, P., et al. The liver tumor segmentation benchmark (lits). CoRR, abs/1901.04056 (2019)
3. Han, Z., Zhang, C., Fu, H., Zhou, J.T.: Trusted multi-view classification. In: International Conference on Learning Representations (2021)
4. He, K., Zhang, X., Ren, S., Sun, J.: Deep residual learning for image recognition. In: Proceedings of the IEEE Conference on Computer Vision and Pattern Recognition (CVPR) (2016)
5. Li, C., et al.: Multi-view mammographic density classification by dilated and attention-guided residual learning. IEEE/ACM Trans. Comput. Biol. Bioinf. **18**(3), 1003–1013 (2020)
6. Setio, A.A.A., et al.: Pulmonary nodule detection in CT images: false positive reduction using multi-view convolutional networks. IEEE Trans. Med. Imaging **35**(5), 1160–1169 (2016)
7. Sun, J., Bi, J., Kranzler, H.R.: Multi-view singular value decomposition for disease subtyping and genetic associations. BMC Genet. **15**(1), 1–12 (2014)
8. Sun, L., Wang, J., Zhijun, H., Yong, X., Cui, Z.: Multi-view convolutional neural networks for mammographic image classification. IEEE Access **7**, 126273–126282 (2019)
9. Vaswani, A., et al.: Attention is all you need. In: Guyon, I., et al., (eds.), Advances in Neural Information Processing Systems, vol. 30. Curran Associates Inc (2017)
10. Xu, S., Chen, Y., Ma, C., Yue, X.: Deep evidential fusion network for image classification. In: Denœux, T., Lefèvre, E., Liu, Z., Pichon, F. (eds.) BELIEF 2021. LNCS (LNAI), vol. 12915, pp. 185–193. Springer, Cham (2021). https://doi.org/10.1007/978-3-030-88601-1_19

11. Xu, X., Zhou, F., et al.: Efficient multiple organ localization in CT image using 3D region proposal network. IEEE Trans. Med. Imaging **38**(8), 1885–1898 (2019)
12. Yang, J., et al.: Reinventing 2D convolutions for 3D images. IEEE J. Biomed. Health Inf. **25**(8), 3009–3018 (2021)
13. Yang, J., Shi, R., Ni, B.: Medmnist classification decathlon: a lightweight automl benchmark for medical image analysis. In: IEEE 18th International Symposium on Biomedical Imaging (ISBI), pp. 191–195 (2021)
14. Yang, J., et al.: Medmnist v2: a large-scale lightweight benchmark for 2D and 3D biomedical image classification. arXiv preprint arXiv:2110.14795 (2021)
15. Zhang, C., Adeli, E., Zhou, T., Chen, X., Shen, D.: Multi-layer multi-view classification for Alzheimer's disease diagnosis. In: Proceedings of the AAAI Conference on Artificial Intelligence, vol. 32 (2018)
16. Zhou, J., Zhang, Q., Zhang, B.: An automatic multi-view disease detection system via collective deep region-based feature representation. Future Gener. Comput. Syst. **115**, 59–75 (2021)
17. Zhu, X., Suk, H.-I., Zhu, Y., Thung, K.-H., Wu, G., Shen, D.: Multi-view classification for identification of Alzheimer's disease. In: Zhou, L., Wang, L., Wang, Q., Shi, Y. (eds.) MLMI 2015. LNCS, vol. 9352, pp. 255–262. Springer, Cham (2015). https://doi.org/10.1007/978-3-319-24888-2_31

Feature Patch Based Attention Model for Dental Caries Classification

Genqiang Ren[1], Yufei Chen[1(✉)], Shuai Qi[2], Yujie Fu[2], and Qi Zhang[2]

[1] College of Electronics and Information Engineering, Tongji University, Shanghai, China
yufeichen@tongji.edu.cn

[2] Department of Endodontics, School and Hospital of Stomatology, Tongji University, Shanghai Engineering Research Center of Tooth Restoration and Regeneration, Shanghai, China

Abstract. Dental caries is a common dental disease. According to statistics, about 90% of adults suffer from dental caries. Therefore, early detection and treatment of dental caries are crucial to dental health. According to the depth of carious lesions, dental caries can be classified into shallow, moderate, and deep caries. Among them, the accurate classification of moderate caries and deep caries is important to making the subsequent treatment plan. Clinically, doctors can make the diagnosis with the help of CBCT images. However, due to the spatial complexity of the 3D volume, the difficulty of labeling the carious lesion, and the insignificant difference between moderate and deep caries, there is still a great challenge to accurately identifying moderate and deep caries. And to the best of our knowledge, there is no study on automatic dental caries classification based on CBCT images. In this paper, we propose a feature patch based attention model to improve the classification accuracy of dental caries in CBCT images. We extract overlapping patches from the 3D feature maps and assign every patch with a corresponding weight computed by adaptive learning to achieve automatic screening of regions that are critical for classification. We collect a real-world dental dataset which includes 167 CBCT scans with moderate caries and 157 CBCT scans with deep caries. A series of experiments demonstrate that our algorithm achieves 92% accuracy on caries classification, which outperforms state-of-the-art methods by a large margin.

Keywords: Dental caries diagnosis · Attention mechanism · Dental cbct

1 Introduction

Dental caries is a multifactorial, dynamic disease that results in net mineral loss of dental hard tissues and a carious lesion [1]. The teeth are composed of three main parts, from the outside to the inside: enamel, dentin, and pulp. Caries start on the enamel surface and progress to the dentin until it affects the whole dentin

Y. Chen et al. (Eds.): CLIP 2022, LNCS 13746, pp. 62–71, 2023.
https://doi.org/10.1007/978-3-031-23179-7_7

layer and finally lead to the inflammation of the pulp. The inflammation of the dental pulp will result in great pain for the patient. As one of the most common chronic dental diseases, caries can occur throughout life, affecting between 60% and 90% of school children and most adults [2,3]. Therefore, early detection and treatment of caries are crucial to dental health.

Corresponding to the depth of the carious lesion, caries has several stages: shallow caries, moderate caries, and deep caries. Different carious lesion depths correspond to different treatment strategies and prognoses. By examining the content of those slices in all three views (Axial, Sagittal, Coronal), clinicians may figure out the carious lesions' depth and the specific relationship between the carious lesions and the pulp in CBCT images, thus formulate further treatment plans. However, this evaluation process is sometimes rather time-consuming and challenging. Clinicians must check hundreds of slices in all three views to acquire comprehensive information about the carious lesions. In addition, CBCT is not as prevalent as periapical radiographs or bitewings in our routine use, leading to the capacity variance among clinicians regarding radiograph diagnosis. Hence, it is of great significance to develop an automated computer-aided system based on CBCT, boosting caries evaluating efficiency on CBCT images and improving the accuracy of diagnosing carious lesions. So far, in the field of dentistry, some deep learning-based of computer-aided diagnosis works have been investigated [4–12]. But, to the best of our knowledge, there is no existing work to classify dental caries in CBCT images. The main technical challenges are as follows: (1) inter-slice variance. The slices of the same CBCT image correspond to different caries categories, for example, some slices belong to moderate caries, and others to deep caries. Labeling all slices in CBCT images is time-consuming and laborious. This limits the use of most 2D CNN models, such as ResNet [13]. (2) low signal-to-noise ratio. The percentage of the carious lesion in the dental CBCT images is tiny, The percentage of the carious lesion in the dental CBCT images is tiny, resulting in the convolution mechanism being unable to capture distinguishing features. Previous studies have shown that caries diagnosis is related to the severity of caries intrusion into the teeth, especially in the dentin region. Hence, directly feeding the whole CBCT image into a deep model usually results in an unsatisfactory diagnosis, as the irrelevant dental region would harm, instead of help, the model's discriminatory power.

The attention mechanism is widely used in deep learning-based models to enhance the influence of task-relevant information while suppressing irrelevant information. Meanwhile, compared to 2D models, 3D models are more popular since they can not only focus on disease-specific volumes but also explore the inter-slice context of those regions, which might be critical to this diagnosis task. In this work, we propose a patch-based attention mechanism that extracts overlapping patches from the 3D feature maps and assigns every patch with a corresponding weight computed by adaptive learning. To enhance the ability to distinguish features of the carious lesion and ignore the irrelevant features, when a patch is a key to the image-level decision, the weight is high; on the contrary, the weight is lower. Inspired by the fact that in diagnosing dental caries, doctors should pay attention to the local information of the lesion area and the global information, which is the relative depth of carious lesions into the dentin, compared to extracting non-overlapping patches strategy, we extract overlapping patches to capture the global information. Meanwhile, compared to the method of extracting patches from the raw image, which will decompose the target into multiple patches, our approach that extracts patches from the 3D feature maps is better for classification by retaining the integrity of the target. The contributions of this paper can be summarized as follows:

- A one-stage dental caries classification framework is proposed. It takes the classification task directly on the source image without additional pre-localiz ation steps.
- A patch attention model is designed based on the 3D feature maps. It adaptively calculates the contribution of each patch and then assigns the corresponding weight so that the lesion region can get more attention for better classification.
- We evaluate the proposed algorithm on a dental dataset containing 324 sets of CBCT images of moderate and deep caries, which are two easily confused diseases in the clinic. Our method has obtained superior results in the task.

2 Related Work

This section briefly introduces previous studies on computer-aided diagnosis methods with 3D medical image data and review attention mechanism related works in medical imaging analysis.

Medical Image Classification. The existing automatic diagnosis in 3D images data are based on segmentation or detection tasks requiring detailed annotations [14,15]. With the auxiliary task, it is possible to first localize the lesion area, which in turn only needs to be fed into a classifier. For example, Xu et. al [14] leveraged the pixel-wise annotations to detect lesions and constructed a classifier based on the segmentation results. To reduce the time and labor cost of manual annotation, 3D medical diagnosis using merely patient-level labels has become a promising alternative. However, due to the low caries signal-to-noise ratio, it is difficult for the conventional CNN to extract more discriminative features when guided by only patient-level labels. Inspired by ViT's [16] idea of cutting the original image into smaller patches to reduce computation, we propose to cut the whole CBCT into multiple patches and filter out the critical patches for classification through an attention mechanism to improve the efficiency of the model. But unlike ViT, which performs non-overlapping cropping on the original image in a way that destroys the integrity of the target (the same object will be divided into multiple patches), we extract patches on the feature space to ensure the integrity of the target.

Attention Mechanism. Motivated by the success of attention in NLP, the attention mechanism has been widely used in the medical imaging analysis domain to enhance the influence of task-relevant information while suppressing irrelevant information [17–19]. Different task-oriented attention modules have been proposed to enhance the features of disease-related regions in images, thus improving the accuracy of classification or segmentation. For instance, Schlemper et. al [17] propose a novel attention gate (AG) model for medical image analysis that automatically learns to focus on target structures of varying shapes and sizes.

Although deep learning-based approaches have performed well in the field of medical image analysis, due to the spatial complexity of the 3D volume, the difficulty of labeling the carious lesion, and the insignificant difference between moderate and deep caries, there is still a great challenge to accurately identifying moderate and deep caries. Considering that attentional mechanisms can enhance task-related features, we explore a patch-based attention mechanism to improve the classification accuracy of dental caries in CBCT images.

3 Methodology

According to the above directions, we construct a framework to perform an automated diagnosis of dental caries using merely patient-level labels in CBCT images. The proposed framework is illustrated in Fig. 1. Compared to ViT [16], instead of extracting patches from raw input images, the CBCT images are fed into a 3D CNN and the patch-level features are obtained through this CNN. Then we assigns every patch with a corresponding weight computed by attention module so that the lesion region can get more attention for better classification.

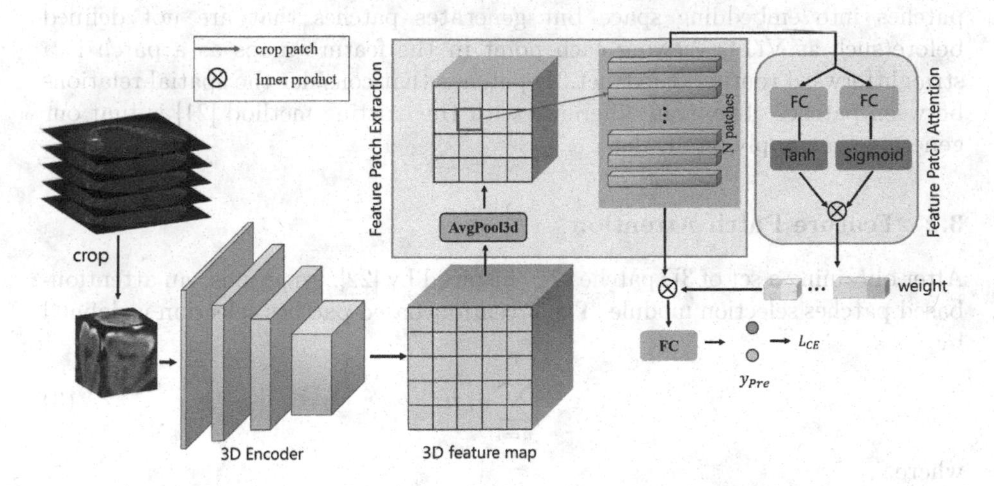

Fig. 1. Illustration of the pipeline of the proposed framework.

3.1 Feature Patch Extraction

Existing popular approaches [20] generally divide the CT/MR images into multiple cubic patches with a fixed size without overlapping. However, such a manner would split the target into different patches, neglecting the spatial and global information. Inspired by the patch extraction in [21], we propose a simple but effective module that extracts patches from feature maps instead of the input image. In addition, to capture the local and global information, we propose extracting overlapping patches. In this manner, each patch has relatively complete semantic information which is essential for the classification task. Generally speaking, given a 3D dental CBCT scan X_i with the shape of $D * H * W$, we can get a 3D feature map $\tilde{X}_i$ using a 3D Encoder. Then, the feature map is fed into an average pooling layer and a new feature map $\hat{X}_i$ is obtained. The shape of $\hat{X}_i$ is $C * D * H * W$, where C, D, H, W represent the channel, depth, high, width, respectively. We view each point of the feature map as a patch with the shape of $C*1$. Hence, in this way, for the given CBCT scan X_i, we extract $N = D*H*W$ patches in total. We define the patch generator operation as ψ, and the patches are as follow:

$$\mathcal{H}_i = \{h_1, h_2, \ldots, h_N\} \tag{1}$$

where N denotes the quantity of patches, $h_i \in \mathbb{R}^{N*C}$. Note that the raw location of corresponding patches on the 3D CBCT scan can be easily derived according to the location of patches on the feature map. Formally, this step can be formulated into:

$$\mathcal{H}_i = \psi(X_i) \tag{2}$$

In conclusion, the patch extraction module in our work not only transforms patches into embedding space but generates patches that are not defined before(such as ViT). Viewing each point in the feature maps as a patch is a straightforward routine to extract 3D patches that consider the spatial relations between patches. The main difference with the existing method [21] is that our generator can apply on 3D data.

3.2 Feature Patch Attention

After obtaining a set of 3D patches $\mathcal{H}_i$, inspired by [22], we propose an attention-based patches selection module. The attention-based patches selection is defined by

$$z = \sum_{n=1}^{N} a_n \boldsymbol{h}_n \tag{3}$$

where,

$$a_n = \frac{\exp\left\{\boldsymbol{w}^\top\left(\tanh\left(\boldsymbol{V}\boldsymbol{h}_n^\top\right) \odot \operatorname{sigm}\left(\boldsymbol{U}\boldsymbol{h}_n^\top\right)\right)\right\}}{\sum_{j=1}^{N} \exp\left\{\boldsymbol{w}^\top\left(\tanh\left(\boldsymbol{V}\boldsymbol{h}_j^\top\right) \odot \operatorname{sigm}\left(\boldsymbol{U}\boldsymbol{h}_j^\top\right)\right)\right\}} \tag{4}$$

where $\boldsymbol{w} \in \mathbb{R}^{N*1}$, $\boldsymbol{V} \in \mathbb{R}^{N*D}$ and $\boldsymbol{U} \in \mathbb{R}^{N*D}$ are trainable parameters. $\odot$ is an element-wise multiplication and sigm(.) is the sigmoid non-linearity. We use the hyperbolic tangent $\tanh(\cdot)$ element-wise non-linearity for proper gradient flow. In simple terms, if a 3D patch has a more significant weight value calculated by the attention module, it means that the semantic features in this patch are essential for the classification task. From another perspective, the weight values calculated by the attention module directly reflect the contribution of each patch extracted in the previous step to the patient-level diagnosis. Therefore, the patch-based attention mechanism gives strong interpretability to the predictions. In summary, let σ_a with parameters θ_{σ_a} represent the attention-based patches selection, this step can be formulated into:

$$z_i = \sigma_a(\mathcal{H}_i) \tag{5}$$

On the feature maps extracted by a 3D Encoder, the patch-based attention is able to filter out task-relevant semantic features. Because of the higher resolution of CBCT images, the number of patches is also quite large, resulting in a surge in weight calculation.

3.3 Loss Function

We train the proposed caries classification model using a patient-level label. The loss function we use in model training based on the cross entropy loss is described as:

$$\mathcal{L}(\mathbf{W}) = -\frac{1}{N}\sum_{n=1}^{N} \log\left(P\left(Y_n \mid \boldsymbol{X}_n; \mathbf{W}\right)\right) \tag{6}$$

where N is the number of images, $P(Y_n \mid \boldsymbol{X}_n; \mathbf{W})$ is the probability of correct prediction for $\boldsymbol{X}_n$, $(\boldsymbol{X}_n, Y_n)$ is the training sample, $\mathbf{W}$ is the parameter of the model.

4 Experiments and Analysis

4.1 Dataset and Settings

Dataset. In this study, we collected a real-world dental dataset comprised of 324 CBCT scans between 2020 and 2022 from Stomatology Hospital. The dataset includes 167 CBCT scans with moderate caries and 157 CBCT scans with deep caries. The random selected dental CBCT image are illustrated in Fig. 2. All images are resampled to 0.1 * 0.1 * 0.1 mm isotropic resolution and labeled by experienced dentists. The splitting of the training set and testing set is according to the patient level. This study and all research were approved and conducted following relevant guidelines/regulations.

Implementation and Details. The framework is implemented using Pytorch 1.9 and trained on a workstation equipped with a NVIDIA GTX 3090 graphics card. During the training process, the model is optimized by Adaptive Moment Estimation(Adam) algorithm with 500 epochs, and the weight decay is $1 * 10^{-4}$. The initial learning rate is 0.0001. For the tooth dataset, 70% of the samples and

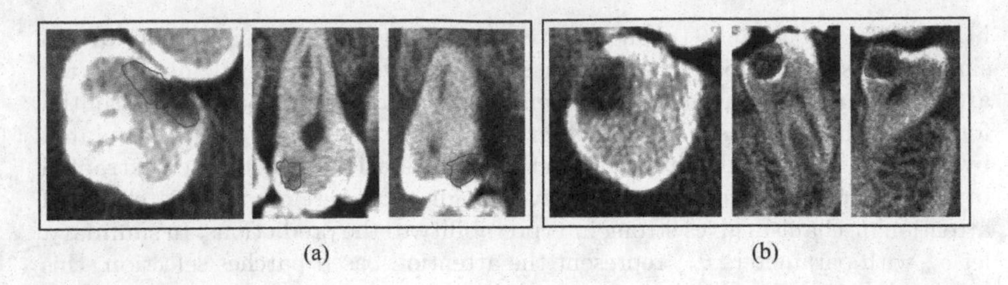

Fig. 2. The visualization of dental CBCT slices from the collected dataset. (a)middle caries (b)deep caries

20% of the samples are respectively selected as the training set and validation set to supervise the training of the model, and 10% of the samples are as the testing set to evaluate the performance.

Evaluation Metrics. In order to verify the effectiveness of the framework, 5-fold cross-validation is adopted, and some evaluation metrics, including $Accuracy = \frac{TP+TN}{TP+TN+FP+FN}$, $F1\ score = \frac{2*Precision*Recall}{Precision+Recall}$, $Recall = \frac{TP}{TP+FN}$, and $Precision = \frac{TP}{TP+FP}$ are used to evaluate the classification performance, where TP, TN, FP, and FN are the number of true positive samples, true negative samples, false positive samples, and false negative samples, respectively.

4.2 Experimental Results

Table 1 shows the result of caries classification on CBCT images. All the used algorithms are achieving promising performance. Among them, our method significantly outperforms the ResNet-18 [13] 3D, Resnet-50 [13] 3D, and GCNet [23] 3D models on almost all metrics.

Table 1. Comparison of classification results of different methods.

	Accuracy	F1-score	Precision	Recall
Resnet-18 [13] 3D	0.7815	0.7746	0.7856	0.7915
Resnet-50 [13] 3D	0.8127	0.7997	0.8100	0.7940
GCNet [23] 3D	0.8235	0.8126	0.8094	0.8035
Proposed	0.9218	0.9193	0.9200	0.9189

It reveals that compared to existing methods, our model is the best in several metrics and can obtain a more interpretable result, as illustrated in Fig. 3. We employed the salience mask of the final trained model to identify the critical

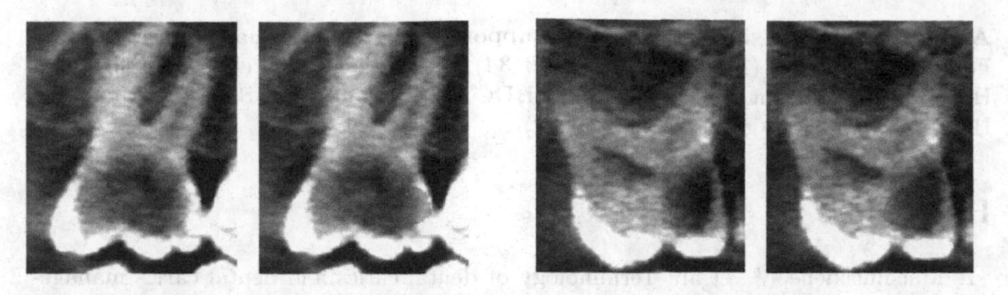

Fig. 3. The visualization of key patches(in red) in dental CBCT image. (Color figure online)

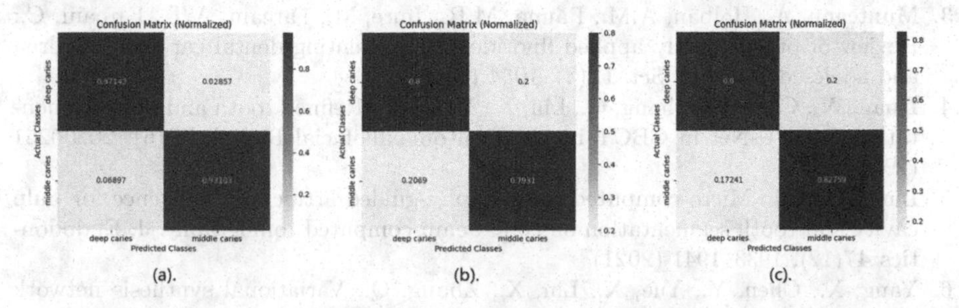

Fig. 4. The confusion matrix of two classes classification: moderate caries and deep caries. (a).Proposed (b). ResNet-50 [13] 3D (c). GCNet [23] 3D

regions for moderate caries vs. deep caries classification. Fig. 4 shows the confusion matrixes of our method, Resnet-50 3D, and GCNet 3D. And our method obtains a balance performance. Comparing ResNet-18 and ResNet-50, two more commonly used backbone models in deep learning, it can be found that simply increasing the model complexity does not significantly improve the accuracy of the model. Comparing GCNet with our model, although both use the attention mechanism, our approach tends to extract features more efficiently, as demonstrated by visualizing the critical patches.

5 Conclusion

Compared with traditional convolution-based mechanisms, our method of patch-based attention model can capture more discriminative features and achieve automatic identification and classification of lesion regions without the aid of auxiliary tasks to localize lesion areas such as segmentation and detection, and the results are interpretable, which can assist clinicians in diagnosis. However, some samples are difficult to distinguish between medium and deep caries solely based on imaging information, and further reference to other clinical information of the patient is needed. In addition, for better clinical application, the current binary classification needs to be extended to four classifications, i.e. normal, superficial, medium and deep caries, which is our future work to be carried out.

Acknowledgements. This work was supported by the National Natural Science Foundation of China (No. 62173252, 61976134), the Clinical Research Plan of Shanghai Hospital Development Center (grant no. SHDC2020CR3058B), the Shanghai Municipal Health Commission (grant no. 202040282).

References

1. Machiulskiene, V., et al.: Terminology of dental caries and dental caries management: consensus report of a workshop organized by ORCA and cariology research group of IADR. Caries Res. **54**(1), 7–14 (2020)
2. Pitts, N.B., et al.: Dental caries. Nat. Rev. Dis. Primers. **3**(1), 1–16 (2017)
3. Munteanu, A., Holban, A.M., Păuna, M.R., Imre, M., Farcaiu, A.T., Farcaiu, C.: Review of professionally applied fluorides for preventing dental caries in children and adolescents. Appl. Sci. **12**(3), 1054 (2022)
4. Duan, W., Chen, Y., Zhang, Q., Lin, X., Yang, X.: Refined tooth and pulp segmentation using U-Net in CBCT image. Dentomaxillofacial Radiol. **50**(6), 20200251 (2021)
5. Lin, X., et al.: Micro-computed tomography-guided artificial intelligence for pulp cavity and tooth segmentation on cone-beam computed tomography. J. Endodontics **47**(12), 1933–1941 (2021)
6. Yang, X., Chen, Y., Yue, X., Lin, X., Zhang, Q.: Variational synthesis network for generating micro computed tomography from cone beam computed tomography. In: 2021 IEEE International Conference on Bioinformatics and Biomedicine (BIBM), pp. 1611–1614. IEEE (2021)
7. Lee, J.H., Kim, D.H., Jeong, S.N., Choi, S.H.: Detection and diagnosis of dental caries using a deep learning-based convolutional neural network algorithm. J. Dent. **77**, 106–111 (2018)
8. Cantu, A.G., et al.: Detecting caries lesions of different radiographic extension on bitewings using deep learning. J. Dent. **100**, 103425 (2020)
9. Casalegno, F., et al.: Caries detection with near-infrared transillumination using deep learning. J. Dent. Res. **98**(11), 1227–1233 (2019)
10. Schwendicke, F., Elhennawy, K., Paris, S., Friebertshäuser, P., Krois, J.: Deep learning for caries lesion detection in near-infrared light transillumination images: a pilot study. J. Dent. **92**, 103260 (2020)
11. Moutselos, K., Berdouses, E., Oulis, C., Maglogiannis, I.: Recognizing occlusal caries in dental intraoral images using deep learning. In: 2019 41st Annual International Conference of the IEEE Engineering in Medicine and Biology Society (EMBC), pp. 1617–1620. IEEE (2019)
12. Liu, L., Xu, J., Huan, Y., Zou, Z., Yeh, S.C., Zheng, L.R.: A smart dental health-IoT platform based on intelligent hardware, deep learning, and mobile terminal. IEEE J. Biomed. Health Inf. **24**(3), 898–906 (2019)
13. He, K., Zhang, X., Ren, S., Sun, J.: Deep residual learning for image recognition. In: Proceedings of the IEEE Conference on Computer Vision and Pattern Recognition, pp. 770–778 (2016)
14. Xu, X., et al.: A deep learning system to screen novel coronavirus disease 2019 pneumonia. Engineering **6**(10), 1122–1129 (2020)
15. Roth, H.R., et al.: Improving computer-aided detection using convolutional neural networks and random view aggregation. IEEE Trans. Med. Imaging **35**(5), 1170–1181 (2015)

16. Dosovitskiy, A., et al.: An image is worth 16x16 words: transformers for image recognition at scale. In: International Conference on Learning Representations (2020)
17. Schlemper, J., et al.: Attention gated networks: learning to leverage salient regions in medical images. Med. Image Anal. **53**, 197–207 (2019)
18. Wang, S., Li, L., Zhuang, X.: AttU-Net: attention U-Net for brain tumor segmentation. In: Crimi, A., Bakas, S. (eds.) International MICCAI Brainlesion Workshop. BrainLes 2021, vol. 12963, pp. 302–311. Springer, Cham (2022)
19. Shen, C., et al.: Attention-guided pancreatic duct segmentation from abdominal CT volumes. In: Oyarzun Laura, C., et al. (eds.) DCL/PPML/LL-COVID19/CLIP -2021. LNCS, vol. 12969, pp. 46–55. Springer, Cham (2021). https://doi.org/10.1007/978-3-030-90874-4_5
20. Gao, X., Qian, Y., Gao, A.: COVID-VIT: Classification of COVID-19 from CT chest images based on vision transformer models. arXiv preprint arXiv:2107.01682 (2021)
21. Yuan, K., Guo, S., Liu, Z., Zhou, A., Yu, F., Wu, W.: Incorporating convolution designs into visual transformers. In: Proceedings of the IEEE/CVF International Conference on Computer Vision, pp. 579–588 (2021)
22. Ilse, M., Tomczak, J., Welling, M.: Attention-based deep multiple instance learning. In: International Conference on Machine Learning, pp. 2127–2136. PMLR (2018)
23. Cao, Y., Xu, J., Lin, S., Wei, F., Hu, H.: GCNet: non-local networks meet squeeze-excitation networks and beyond. In: Proceedings of the IEEE/CVF International Conference on Computer Vision Workshops (2019)

Conditional Domain Adaptation Based on Initial Distribution Discrepancy for EEG Emotion Recognition

Mohan Zhao[1(✉)], Lu Pang[1(✉)], Yan Lu[1], Fei Xie[1], Zhenghao He[1], Xiaoliang Gong[1], and Anthony George Cohn[1,2]

[1] College of Electronics and Information Engineering, Tongji University, Shanghai, China
{1951854,gxllshsh}@tongji.edu.cn
[2] University of Leeds, Leeds, UK

Abstract. How to integrate data in different feature spaces and distributions is a research hotspot in EEG-based emotion recognition. A novel source-domain adaptation strategy based on initial distribution differences for EEG emotion recognition is proposed, which selects several source domains that are most similar to the target domain for domain adaptation. Compared to the 'source-target pair' domain adaptation method using all source domains, this method improves accuracy by up to 10% and reduces computation time by up to 43%, based on the SEED-III and SEED-IV datasets.

Keywords: Emotion recognition · EEG · Transfer learning · Domain adaptation

1 Introduction

Emotions play an important role in the life of human-beings. EEG signals are one way to recognize people's emotions by machines [1,2]. The acquisition of EEG signals is affected by many factors such as individuals and equipment, resulting in different feature spaces and distributions across the data [3,4]. In practical application scenarios, it is usually required to use the original data to predict the emotional state of a new individual from their EEG signals. These cross-subject and cross-experiment data will result in low accuracy if trained and tested using a traditional machine learning model [5]. Therefore, how to integrate data for effective learning is a focus of research in this area.

Supported by National-level Computer and Information Technology Experimental Teaching Demonstration Center (0800120010) and National Innovation and Entrepreneurship Program for Undergraduates of Tongji University 2022 (Practice and Research of Artificial Intelligence Algorithm for Emotion Recognition in Chinese Traditional Music).

Y. Chen et al. (Eds.): CLIP 2022, LNCS 13746, pp. 72–81, 2023.
https://doi.org/10.1007/978-3-031-23179-7_8

An important assumption that traditional machine learning relies on is that training data and future data must have the same feature space and distribution [6], but in many practical application scenarios, this assumption cannot be satisfied [7]. One solution is to introduce transfer learning in which data in the source learning system constitutes the source domain, and data in target learning system constitutes the target domain [8].

Domain Adaptation is a method of transfer learning, which is suitable for situations where the distributions of data features in the source and target domains are different [9]. This method inputs the data of the two domains into a feature transformer, thus changing these data into a new feature space. The distribution difference between the source domain and the target domain in this new feature space is then calculated by a specific distribution similarity criterion. The adaptation process is to train the feature extractor so that the distribution difference between the two target domains is as small as possible after transformation.

In this paper, a source-domain adaptation strategy based on initial distribution differences for EEG emotion recognition is proposed. This strategy does not use all source domains for domain adaptation, but selects those source domains that are most similar to the target domain for domain adaptation. The similarity criterion between target and source is the distribution difference without domain adaptation feature transformation. The target domain and each source domain respectively form a 'source domain-target domain pair' for domain adaptation. Based on the SEED-III and SEED-IV datasets, we test the accuracy and computation time for the proposed method using the chosen metric, and make comparisons with the original method.

2 Materials

Domain adaptation has been frequently used in the training of EEG-related models in recent years. Chai et al. [10] proposed a fast domain adaptation strategy that integrates marginal and conditional distributions into a single in a unified framework. Lin and Jung [11] explored a conditional transfer learning framework for sentiment classification by selectively applying data with similar feature spaces by evaluating the transferability of each sample. They use ReliefF [12] to form a feature space and use Pearson's correlation coefficient as an indicator of source domain selection, which, however, is not a specific strategy. Chen et al. [13] proposed a multi-source marginal distribution adaptation strategy (MSMDA), which pairs the target domain and each source domain one by one to form a 'source domain-target domain pair' for domain adaptation. The problem of information loss may be caused by merging all source domains into one source domain. However, using all source domains may lead to negative transfer due to too large gaps between some source and target domains.

Li-Ming et al. [14] devised a methodology called plug-and-play adaptation for cross-subject EEG-based emotion recognition, which can be used to enhance user experience and make EEG-based affective computing applications more practicable. Jinpeng et al. [15] proposed a multisource transfer learning method, where existing persons are sources, and the new person is the target. In the work of Dongdong et al. [16], a multiple source domain adaptation method is proposed to learn fault-discriminative but working condition-invariant features from raw vibration signals. Different known working conditions are assigned different weights, on the basis of their distributional similarities to the target working condition. Zirui et al. [17] compared two public datasets DEAP and SEED used in domain adapation, based on which in this paper SEED is chosen for its coverage.

The datasets used in this paper are SEED-III [18] and SEED-IV [19]. SEED is a series of datasets for EEG sentiment analysis, which uses discrete sentiment classification as labels, with three sentiment labels in SEED-III and 4 in SEED-IV. 15 subjects participated in the data collection. In order to ensure the universality of the data, each dataset is divided into three sessions, each session representing data taken in a period of time. There are 15 trails in a session. The device collected EEG data from 62 channels (electrodes) of the subjects (Fig. 1).

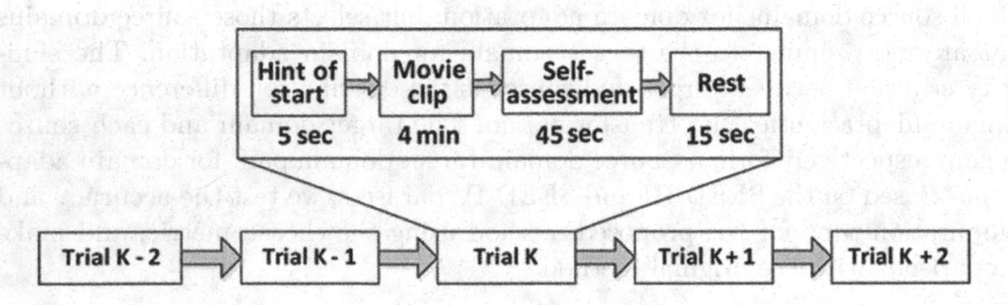

Fig. 1. The data collection process within a trail. In a trail, subjects watch a 4-min movie clip, and the emotional label corresponding to the 4-min EEG data is determined by the type of movie clip.

The collected data is firstly processed by down-sampling 200 Hz and filtered at 0 75 Hz, and then mapped to five commonly used frequency bands through Fourier transform. Finally, the differential entropy is used to process the data sequence. The relevant literature [20] proves that the differential entropy is more suitable for EEG data than other feature extraction methods.

3 Methods

Inspired by the work of Lin and Jung [11] and Chen [13], we propose two hypotheses: (1) conditionally selecting several source domains whose initial distribution is most similar to the target domain, and using these source domains, ideal classification results can be achieved; (2) since the contribution of each source domain to model training is different. The more similar a source domain and the target domain are in the initial distribution, the better the effect of using this source domain for domain adaptation, and the greater the accuracy of the model.

A series of experiments were conducted to test these hypotheses using SEED-III and SEED-IV, thus obtaining and validating a conditional source domain selection strategy based on initial distribution differences.

The model used is an improved version of MSMDA [13]. In Fig. 2, each source and target domain is the EEG data of a certain subject. Before performing domain adaptation, it is necessary to calculate the initial distribution difference (dist. discrepancy) between each source domain and the target domain. The blue source field in the figure indicates that the difference is acceptable, and the red one indicates it is not. The remaining domains including source and target are then sent to Common Feature Extractor to extract their common features. Source domains are paired one by one with the target domain and enter the Domain-specific Feature Extractor, where the distribution difference between the two is calculated as part of the loss function (dist. loss). Then, the output of each DSFE is fed into the corresponding domain-specific classifier. The magnitudes of the difference between results of these classifiers are also used as part of the loss function (disc. loss). Finally for each DSC, the difference (cls. loss) between their output and the actual label is calculated. The final output of the model is the average of all DSC outputs.

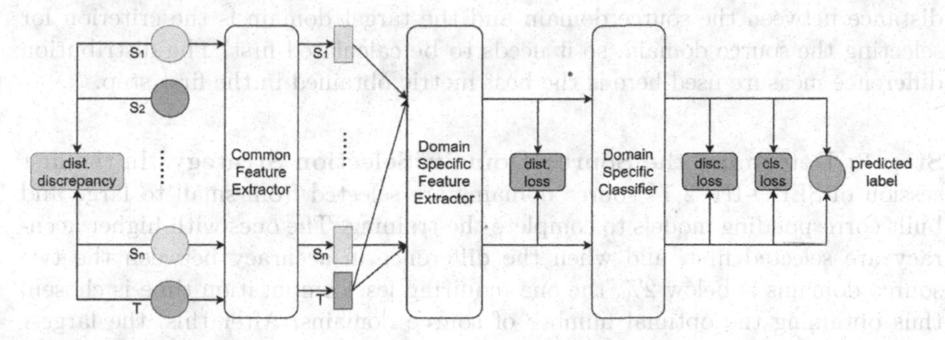

Fig. 2. The structure of the proposed model. The main difference from MSMDA is that the initial distribution difference between the source domain and the target domain is calculated before entering the model, thereby eliminating those source domains with large differences.

Step 1: Finding the Best Distribution Difference Metric. Currently, the most commonly used metric in domain adaptation is the Maximum Mean Discrepancy (MMD). The formula is as follows:

$$MMD(p, q, F) = \left\| \frac{1}{m} \sum_{i=1}^{n} f(x_i) - \frac{1}{n} \sum_{j=1}^{m} f(y_j) \right\|_H \quad (1)$$

However, the calculation of MMD needs to use a Gaussian kernel function, and the calculation process is relatively cumbersome. Note that the data in the source and target domains in the model have been transformed by DFE before dist. Loss is calculated. Therefore, the mean difference of norm 1 can be calculated directly on the transformed data (Mean Discrepancy, MD-L1). Its formula is as follows:

$$MD(p, q) = \left\| \frac{1}{n} \sum_{i=1}^{n} x_i - \frac{1}{m} \sum_{j=1}^{m} y_j \right\|_1 \tag{2}$$

It has also been proposed [21] that K-L Divergence (KLD) can be used to measure the distribution difference: the smaller the value of KLD, the more similar the two distributions are. KLD is defined as follows:

$$D_{KL}(p\|q) = \sum_{i=1}^{n} p(x_i) \log \frac{p(x_i)}{q(x_i)} \tag{3}$$

In order to choose the best metric, three metrics are used to compare the accuracy and computation time of the model. These three metrics are used in the model as dist. discrepancy and dist. loss.

Step 2: Calculate the Initial Variance of the Distribution. The initial distance between the source domain and the target domain is the criterion for selecting the source domain, so it needs to be calculated first. The distribution difference measure used here is the best metric obtained in the first step.

Step 3: Determine the Source Domain Selection Strategy. In the first session of SEED-III, 2 14 source domains are selected from small to large and built corresponding models to complete the training. The ones with higher accuracy are selected first, and when the difference in accuracy between the two source domains is below 2%, the one requiring less computation time is chosen, thus obtaining the optimal number of source domains. After this, the largest distances (i.e. distribution differences) of these source domains relative to the target domain can be obtained (d_{max}), and the average distance is d_{avg}. A ratio $p = d_{max}/d_{avg}$ between the largest distance and the average distance can be used to determine the optimal source domain selection strategy: for a new target domain, set its average distance to all source domains to be d'_{avg}, a predicted distance threshold $d'_{max} = p * d'_{avg}$ can be obtained; all source domains with distances less than this threshold can be selected for domain adaptation toward the target domain.

Step 4: Verify Source Domain Selection Policy. To validate our proposed conditional source domain strategy, data from other sessions of SEED-III and all sessions of SEED-IV is used. The accuracy and time-consuming between proposed method and MSMDA are compared [13].

4 Results

4.1 The Best Distribution Difference Metric

Table 1. The average and variance of the accuracy and calculation time of the three indicators

Metric	Average accuracy/%	Standard deviation	Average computation time/s	Standard deviation
MMD	82.87	8.56	2745	7
MD-L1	83.58	6.61	2606	6
KLD	74.12	8.11	2629	5

Table 1 shows the accuracy and calculation time corresponding to the three metrics in the first session of SEED-III with different subjects as the target domain. The remaining 14 subjects were used as the source domains. It can be seen that the accuracy of MMD and MD-L1 is comparable, and that of MD-L1 has less fluctuation among subjects. Among the three metrics, the computation time of MD-L1 is the lowest, KLD the second, and MMD the highest. Considering both accuracy and calculation time, MD-L1 is the best. Subsequent experiments will use MD-L1 as a measure of distributional differences.

4.2 Source Domain Selection Strategy

Table 2. The optimal number of source domains and related data for each subject

Subject number	Optimal number	The farthest distance	Average distance	p value
0	11	0.0547	0.0422	1.30
1	10	0.0328	0.0230	1.42
2	7	0.0145	0.0228	0.64
3	14	0.0871	0.0319	2.73
4	14	0.0531	0.0256	2.07
5	10	0.0357	0.0353	1.01
6	11	0.0505	0.0243	2.08
7	2	0.0230	0.0631	0.36
8	7	0.0438	0.0418	1.05
9	11	0.0531	0.0411	1.29
10	9	0.0316	0.0253	1.25
11	5	0.0076	0.0228	0.33
12	10	0.0390	0.0384	1.01
13	12	0.0475	0.0228	2.08
14	5	0.0078	0.0225	0.35

Table 2 shows the optimal number of source domains and related information. The p-value is the ratio of the largest source domain distance to the average domain distance. At the optimal number of source domains, most subjects had p-values between 1 and 1.5. Therefore, when p = 1.5, that is, when the largest distance of the selected source domain is 1.5 times the average distance from the target domain to all source domains, the accuracy and computation time reach the best balance. Combined with the selection order of the source domain, the optimal conditional source domain selection strategy can be obtained as Algorithm 1.

Algorithm 1. Optimal Conditional Source Domain Selection Strategy

Inputs:target domain T,source domains S_1,S_2,...,S_n

(1) Calculate the distance between each source domain and target domain $d(T, S_i)$,with the metric $MD - L1$.

(2) Sort the source domains according to $d(T, S_i)$ from small to large, and set the order of the source domain after sorting as $S_{d_1}, S_{d_2}, ..., S_{d_n}$.

(3) Suppose the set of selected source domains is $\mathcal{S} = S_(d_1)$,the average distance from the target domain to all source domains is $S_avg, i = 2$.

(4) if $d(T, S_(d_i)) \leq d_avg \times 1.5$, add $S_(d_i)$to $\mathcal{S}$,$i = i + 1$, repeat this step,otherwise end.

Outputs: set of source domains for domain adaptation $\mathcal{S}$

4.3 Verifying the Source Domain Selection Strategy

Table 3. Average accuracy of source domain selection strategy and original method

Data	The optimal strategy/%	The original method/%
SEED-III session2	77.49	77.21
SEED-III session3	80.09	78.80
SEED-IV session1	55.00	54.79
SEED-IV session2	62.43	55.79
SEED-IV session3	61.65	55.39

Table 4. Average computation time of source domain selection strategy and original method

Data	The optimal strategy/s	The original method/s
SEED-III session2	1963	2890
SEED-III session3	1643	2886
SEED-IV session1	531	697
SEED-IV session2	493	689
SEED-IV session3	466	690

In terms of accuracy (as shown in Table 3), the source domain selection strategy is slightly higher than MSMDA, and this advantage is more obvious in SEED-IV.

In terms of computation time (as shown in Table 4), the source domain selection strategy is greatly reduced compared to MSMDA. Validation experiments show that the conditional source domain selection strategy can achieve higher accuracy with a smaller number of source domains, and the required computation time is also greatly reduced.

5 Discussion

Effectiveness of Source Domain Selection Strategy. It can be concluded from the experiment that for most subjects, the peak of the accuracy rate does not appear when the number of source domains is 14, indicating that negative transfer occurred. Table 3 shows that the source domain selection strategy has a certain improvement in accuracy compared to the original method. Besides, since the conditional selection strategy reduces the usage of source domains, the scale of the model is also reduced, so the overall computation time is also significantly lower than the original method.

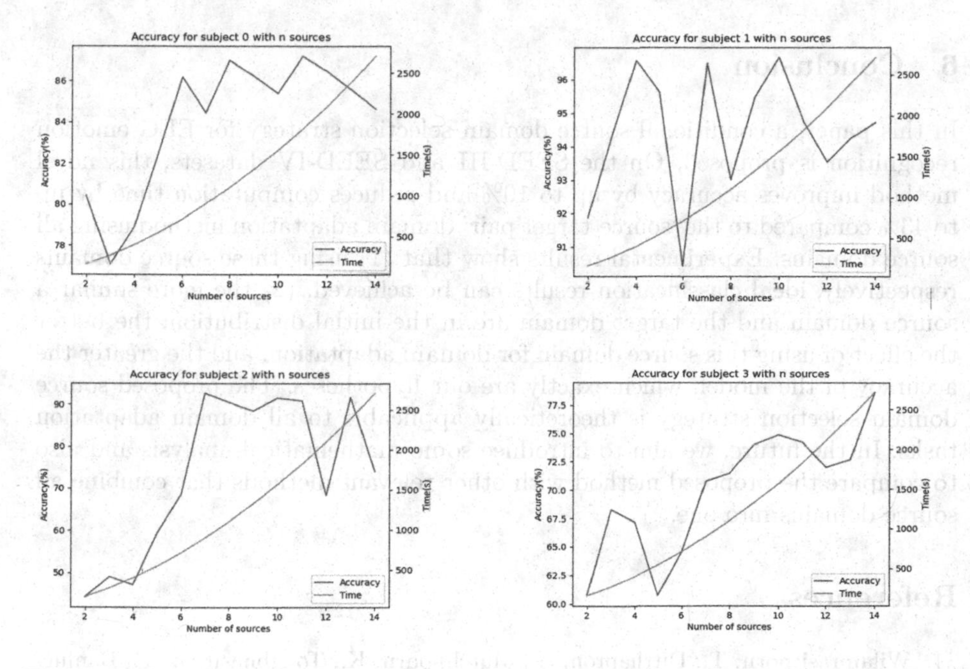

Fig. 3. The trend of accuracy and computation time of the top 4 subjects in the first session of SEED-III with number of source domains. The abscissa is the number of source domains, the blue line the accuracy, and the orange line the computation time. (Color figure online)

Extension of Source Domain Selection Strategy in Other Fields. The proposed source domain selection strategy is theoretically applicable to all domain adaptation tasks. As machine learning technology gradually penetrates into various applications, more tasks with data heterogeneity and data scarcity will appear in the future, and the proposed method is expected to improve the performance of machine learning models in those tasks.

Limitations of Source Domain Selection Strategy. For a new target domain (subject), the number of source domains to select is related to the optimal number of source domains for the existing data. In fact, it can be seen from Fig. 3 that the accuracy rate with the number of source domains is not a single peak, indicating that the initial distribution difference between source and target cannot completely determine the contribution of the source domain to the model. In order to obtain better source domain selection criteria, some mathematical analysis may need to be introduced. In validation experiments, only comparison with MSMDA is made, which can only show that the proposed method outperforms the 'source-target pair' full-source domain adaptation method. To further evaluate our method, it is necessary to compare the proposed method with those methods that combine all source domains into one.

6 Conclusion

In this paper, a conditional source domain selection strategy for EEG emotion recognition is proposed. On the SEED-III and SEED-IV datasets, this novel method improves accuracy by up to 10% and reduces computation time by up to 43% compared to the 'source-target pair' domain adaptation method using all source domains. Experimental results show that (1) using these source domains respectively, ideal classification results can be achieved. (2) the more similar a source domain and the target domain are in the initial distribution, the better the effect of using this source domain for domain adaptation, and the greater the accuracy of the model, which exactly are our hypotheses. The proposed source domain selection strategy is theoretically applicable to all domain adaptation tasks. In the future, we aim to introduce some mathematical analysis and also to compare the proposed method with other relevant methods that combine all source domains into one.

References

1. Wilaiprasitporn, T., Ditthapron, A., Matchaparn, K., Tongbuasirilai, T., Banluesombatkul, N., Chuangsuwanich, E.: Affective EEG-based person identification using the deep learning approach. IEEE Trans. Cogn. Develop. Syst. **12**(3), 486–496 (2020)
2. Alarcão, S.M., Fonseca, M.J.: Emotions recognition using EEG signals: a survey. IEEE Trans. Affect. Comput. **10**(3), 374–393 (2019)
3. Wan, Z., Yang, R., Huang, M., Zeng, N., Liu, X.: A review on transfer learning in EEG signal analysis. Neurocomputing **421**, 1–14 (2021). https://www.sciencedirect.com/science/article/pii/S0925231220314223

4. Rahman, M.M., et al.: Recognition of human emotions using EEG signals: a review. Comput. Biol. Med. **136**, 104696 (2021). https://www.sciencedirect.com/science/article/pii/S001048252100490X
5. Cimtay, Y., Ekmekcioglu, E.: Investigating the use of pretrained convolutional neural network on cross-subject and cross-dataset EEG emotion recognition. Sensors **20**(7), 2034 (2020)
6. Csurka, G.: A comprehensive survey on domain adaptation for visual applications. In: Csurka, G. (ed.) Domain Adaptation in Computer Vision Applications. ACVPR, pp. 1–35. Springer, Cham (2017). https://doi.org/10.1007/978-3-319-58347-1_1
7. Pan, S.J., Yang, Q.: A survey on transfer learning. IEEE Trans. Knowl. Data Eng. **22**(10), 1345–1359 (2010)
8. Wang, J., et al.: Generalizing to unseen domains: a survey on domain generalization. IEEE Trans. Knowl. Data Eng., 1 (2022)
9. Yan, K., Kou, L., Zhang, D.: Learning domain-invariant subspace using domain features and independence maximization. IEEE Trans. Cybern. **48**(1), 288–299 (2018)
10. Chai, X., et al.: A fast, efficient domain adaptation technique for cross-domain electroencephalography (EEG)-based emotion recognition. Sensors **17**(5), 1014 (2017)
11. Lin, Y.-P., Jung, T.-P.: Improving EEG-based emotion classification using conditional transfer learning. Front. Hum. Neurosci. **11**, 334 (2017)
12. Robnik-Šikonja, M., Kononenko, I.: Theoretical and empirical analysis of Relieff and RRelieff. Mach. Learn. **53**(1), 23–69 (2003)
13. Chen, H., Jin, M., Li, Z., Fan, C., Li, J., He, H.: MS-MDA: multisource marginal distribution adaptation for cross-subject and cross-session EEG emotion recognition. Front. Neurosci. **15** (2021)
14. Zhao, L.M., Yan, X., Lu, B.L.: Plug-and-play domain adaptation for cross-subject EEG-based emotion recognition. In: Proceedings of the AAAI Conference on Artificial Intelligence, vol. 35, no. 1, pp. 863–870 (2021)
15. Li, J., Qiu, S., Shen, Y.-Y., Liu, C.-L., He, H.: Multisource transfer learning for cross-subject EEG emotion recognition. IEEE Trans. Cybern. **50**(7), 3281–3293 (2020)
16. Wei, D., Han, T., Chu, F., Zuo, M.J.: Weighted domain adaptation networks for machinery fault diagnosis. Mech. Syst. Signal Process. **158**, 107744 (2021). https://www.sciencedirect.com/science/article/pii/S0888327021001394
17. Lan, Z., Sourina, O., Wang, L., Scherer, R., Müller-Putz, G.R.: Domain adaptation techniques for EEG-based emotion recognition: a comparative study on two public datasets. IEEE Trans. Cogn. Dev. Syst. **11**(1), 85–94 (2019)
18. Zheng, W.-L., Lu, B.-L.: Investigating critical frequency bands and channels for EEG-based emotion recognition with deep neural networks. IEEE Trans. Auton. Ment. Dev. **7**(3), 162–175 (2015)
19. Zheng, W.-L., Liu, W., Lu, Y., Lu, B.-L., Cichocki, A.: EmotionMeter: a multimodal framework for recognizing human emotions. IEEE Trans. Cybern. **49**(3), 1110–1122 (2019)
20. Duan, R.N., Zhu, J.Y., Lu, B.L.: Differential entropy feature for EEG-based emotion classification. In: 2013 6th International IEEE/EMBS Conference on Neural Engineering (NER), pp. 81–84. IEEE (2013)
21. Do, M., Vetterli, M.: Wavelet-based texture retrieval using generalized gaussian density and kullback-leibler distance. IEEE Trans. Image Process. **11**(2), 146–158 (2002)

Automated Cone and Vessel Analysis in Adaptive Optics Like Retinal Images for Clinical Diagnostics Support

Anna-Sophia Hertlein[1,2(✉)], Stefan Wesarg[1], Jessica Schmidt[2], Benjamin Boche[2], Norbert Pfeiffer[3], and Juliane Matlach[3]

[1] Fraunhofer Institute for Computer Graphics Research IGD, Darmstadt, Germany
anna-sophia.hertlein@igd.fraunhofer.de

[2] Interactive Graphics System Group GRIS, Technical University of Darmstadt, Darmstadt, Germany

[3] Department of Ophthalmology, University Medical Center Mainz, Mainz, Germany

Abstract. Today, modern non-invasive Adaptive Optics (AO) imaging enables visualization of cone photoreceptors and vessels on a cellular level. High Magnification Module (HMM) images strongly resemble AO images and can be acquired fast and cost-effectly in clinical routine. Manual examination of those images, however, is tedious and time-consuming. Therefore, methods are needed to automatically analyse HMM images to facilitate the work of ophthalmologists. In this work an automatic cone detection method is presented that robustly detects cones in these images of both healthy and glaucoma patients. In addition, a vessel segmentation algorithm is provided to mask vessels during cone detection and additionally provide the ophthalmologist with vessel diameters that aid in monitoring ocular and cardiovascular diseases. The results on the given data are comparable to the performance of a trained expert and the methods are already being used in clinical practice.

Keywords: Retina analysis · Cone detection · Cone density · Vessel segmentation · Adaptive optics · High magnification module

1 Introduction

Parameters such as cone density or vessel diameter can play an important role in the diagnosis and monitoring of ocular and cardiovascular diseases. Many retinal diseases are associated with the loss of various retinal cells such as cone photoreceptors or their functionality. Analysis of the appearance of retinal vessels can be helpful in diagnosing cardiovascular diseases such as hypertension or diabetes. Today, with non-invasive imaging technologies like Adaptive Optics (AO) it is possible to visualize cone photoreceptors at cellular level. While AO offers very good image quality, the devices are usually very expensive and often require long image acquisition times. The High Magnification Module (HMM) was developed by Heidelberg Engineering and is used as an add-on lens for

Y. Chen et al. (Eds.): CLIP 2022, LNCS 13746, pp. 82–90, 2023.
https://doi.org/10.1007/978-3-031-23179-7_9

their Spectralis®-OCT. HMM creates images very close to AO and makes them available in clinical routine, simplifying the workflow of ophthalmologists for diagnosis and disease monitoring. However, manual segmentation of vessels or counting of cones in these images is tedious and time-consuming. Therefore, methods are needed that automate these processes.

To acquire cone density, first the individual cones have to be detected and quantified. Cone detection algorithms in AO images can be roughly divided into supervised learning, unsupervised learning and classical image processing methods. Supervised learning methods have achieved good results on AO images but require labeled training data as ground truth, which is not always provided and laborious to create [3,4]. Unsupervised learning methods mainly concentrate on counting cones in specific AO images with a much higher spatial resolution [1,2] and are not directly applicable to HMM images. One of the most popular methods is that of Li and Roorda [6] who use that cones appear as bright dots on a darker background in AO images. They apply a regional maximum search to find the individual cones. A local maximum based approach is also used in [8] to estimate cone density in HMM images. They first apply a high-pass filter to enhance the visibility of cones. However, they had to carefully adjust the filter parameters in a trial-and-error process for healthy and unhealthy objects. Furthermore, the results overestimate the amount of cones compared to the manual detections made by experts and they completely avoid regions with blood vessels. One drawback of these intensity based methods is that they also identify cones inside blood vessels, where no cones should be detected. In [7] the authors propose a segmentation algorithm for vessels in AO images to mask out segmented vessels. They use a vesselness filter, thresholding and region growing to obtain a vessel mask. This method though does not seem to be too robust and is relatively slow compared to a modern model-based segmentation. At present the most widely used and best performing image segmentation methods are Neural Networks (NNs). U-Net [9] is a widely used NN that performs well in medical image segmentation tasks and generates good results even on small datasets.

There are many cone detection methods that work on high resolution example images where individual cones are easily recognizable, but no approaches yet that perform well on low resolution HMM images from clinical routine. In contrast to that we provide methods for automatic analysis of HMM images which are of lower resolution and contain more noise and artifacts. This makes adjustment of the previously presented approaches necessary. We introduce methods for both robust automatic cone density and vessel diameter estimation. The proposed methods provide support for diagnosis and monitoring of retinal and vascular diseases. They facilitate the work of ophthalmologists and are already being used in a clinical environment.

2 Methods

In this section we present our methods for automatic analysis of HMM retinal images. The provided methods combine multiple analysis and visualization methods to allow clinicians to automatically calculate vessel diameter, measure and view global and local cone density in HMM images of the retina. A method is presented to detect cones to determine cone density in images of both healthy patients and patients with glaucoma. Like [10] we first perform bias field correction as a preprocessing step to create a more uniformly illuminated image. Similar to previous methods we exploit the bright, blob like appearance of cones. Blob detection with Laplacian-of-Gaussian (LoG) first finds suitable candidates, which are then further classified using a thresholding procedure and non-maximum suppression. To remove cone candidates inside vessels we pick up the idea of [7] and perform a vessel segmentation. For this purpose, we created labeled data in a semi-supervised process and trained a U-Net [9] for automatic segmentation. The resulting vessel masks are used both for cone detection to exclude falsely detected cones inside vessels as well as for vessel diameter assessment. Additionally to global cone counting and global cone density determination we also provide cone density maps that show the density of cones around each pixel.

2.1 Requirements and Data Specifics

The methods have been developed for clinical routine. The ophthalmologists acquire HMM images of the retina during clinical examinations with a Spectralis® (Heidelberg Engineering). This innovative image acquisition system offers the possibility to take images of the human retina in everyday clinical routine that are to a great extent comparable to AO images. One requirement is a robust cone detection on images in clinical routine. No cones should be detected within vessels and the method should work on images of healthy patients as well as on patients with retinal diseases diagnosed. However, the resolution of HMM images is somewhat lower than in AO images. Also many of the images contain motion blur and noise, which further complicates the detection of cones. Therefore, previously known methods cannot be applied directly and must be adapted to work on HMM images. Additionally to cone detection, the ophthalmologists want to measure the vessel diameter to gain further insights into the health status of the patients and investigate correlations between cone functionality loss and loss of ganglion cells and nerve fibers.

2.2 Vessel Segmentation and Analysis

Vessel segmentation serves two purposes here. First, vessel masks are used during cone detection to exclude cones that are falsely detected within vessels. Secondly, vessel diameters can provide clues to common vascular diseases such as hypertension or diabetes. In glaucoma patients, in areas of ganglion cells loss, blood vessels also recede.

To obtain a fast and reliable segmentation of retina vessels, we trained a NN. We used a semi-automatic process to create labeled training data where we first applied a filtering pipeline with a vesselness filter and some morphological filters, then manually corrected the resulting segmentation masks. The created masks were confirmed by an expert and used to train a U-Net [9] instance.

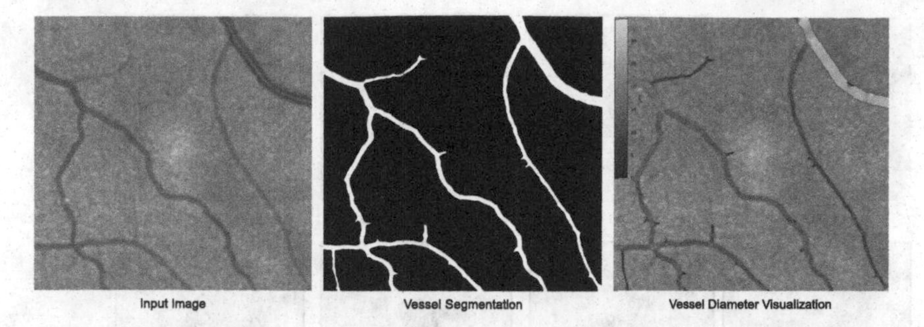

Fig. 1. Vessel diameter determination. On the left the original image, in the middle the vessels segmented with the trained U-Net, and on the right the color-coded vessel diameter

The trained U-Net model is then being used to automatically segment vessels in HMM images. From the automatically created vessel segmentations we calculate the diameter at every pixel along each vessel using a standard skeletonization based approach. To visualize vessel diameters they are represented by a color-coding (see Fig. 1).

2.3 Cone Analysis

To determine the cone density in HMM images, first a detection of individual cones in the input images is performed. The image intensity values are first balanced by a bias field correction before cone candidates are determined with a LoG blob detection. In two post-processing steps first an automatic thresholding is performed to discard dark candidates. Afterwards as explained in Sect. 2.2 we use a U-Net to segment the vessels to sort out cone candidates that are incorrectly located inside vessels. The last step is a non maximum suppression to find the maximum of cone candidates that are very close to each other. Figure 2 shows the whole cone detection pipeline.

Bias Field Correction. In some input images, the illumination of the image varies locally, making intensity-based cone detection difficult. To compensate for this before further processing, a bias field correction is performed using the method proposed by [3].

LoG Blob Detection. The bias field corrected image is then used to find cone candidates. In contrast to [6] who use a local maxima search to detect cones, we apply the Laplacian of Gaussian (LoG) blob detection method at multiple scales, a blob detection method that leads to very accurate results. Blobs in this context are defined as regions in the image with an approximately constant intensity that is brighter than the surrounding area.

Vessel Masking. After the first detection step, there are still many false cone candidates that we want to remove. Most of them are located inside vessels.

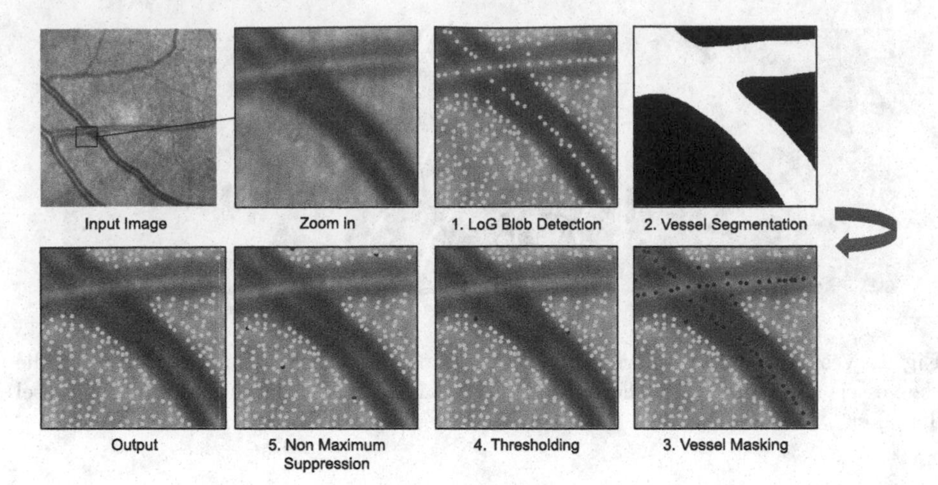

Fig. 2. Cone detection pipeline. The method is executed on the entire image. Zoomed in on a small section for better visibility of the cones.

These candidates can be blood cells or endothelial cells of the vessel wall. The vessel segmentation explained in Sect. 2.2 is used for masking.

Thresholding. Furthermore, we only want to detect active cones which are not damaged. Active cones orient towards the light and thus have a bright appearance. Therefore we want to remove cone candidates with a rather dark appearance. For this purpose, an automatic thresholding step is applied. To automatically determine the optimal threshold we use the well-known Otsu thresholding method. All cone candidates whose intensity value falls below the automatically determined threshold are filtered out.

Non Maximum Suppression. In the last step, groups of cone candidates are identified, which are too close to each other to belong to different cones. For this purpose, a mask with every cone candidate is created. Then a circle with a radius of 2 pixels is drawn on each determined cone candidate pixel. This value corresponds to a cone diameter of about 4 μm which is on the lower end of cone size, which ranges from about 3 μm in the fovea to 10 μm diameter outside the fovea [5]. From this mask, all connected components are determined and for each connected component a group with all cones that belong to it is created. In the next step, in all groups that contain more than one cone candidate, the intensity values of all cone candidate pixels are compared. Only the candidate with the highest intensity value is kept and the others are discarded. The result of this last step is the final outcome of our cone detection algorithm. The detected cones are then counted to obtain the overall cone density of the image.

Cone Density Maps. To obtain a visualization of the local density distribution of the cones in different image regions, additional cone density maps are created. For this purpose, a cone mask image is created with each cone location having the

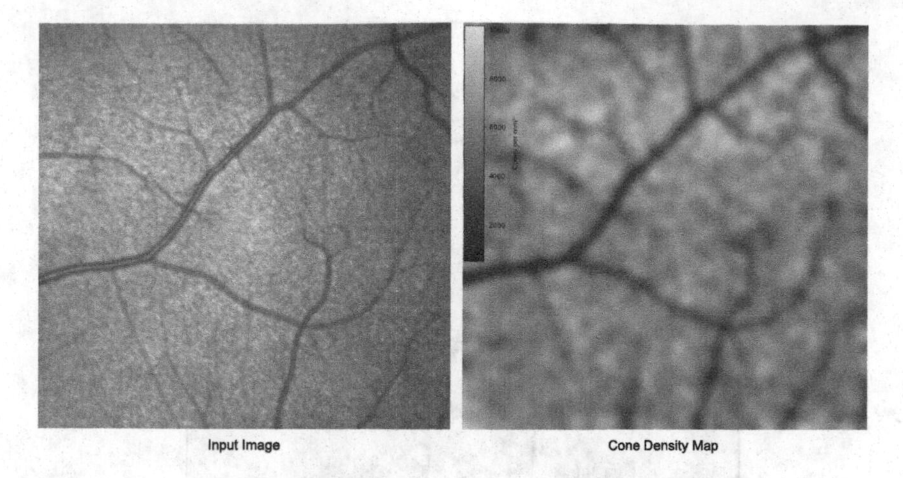

Fig. 3. Cone density map of an HMM image

value 1. Then a Gaussian blur filter is applied with a kernel size of 111×111 px and a standard deviation of 20 px. The result is a map that includes the neighbourhood and shows a local cone density distribution for each pixel. The density values are transferred to a color scheme for better visualization (see Fig. 3).

3 Evaluation and Results

Data. The image data was provided by the department of ophthalmology of the University Hospital Mainz. HMM images were taken from a total of 53 patients, 33 with glaucoma and 20 healthy subjects. Nine images were taken in the same pattern around the macula for each patient (see Fig. 4), which results in a total of 477 images. The images have a size of approximately 1534×1534 px, which corresponds to approximately $1.61\,\text{mm} \times 1.61\,\text{mm}$ or $2.6\,\text{mm}^2$. For U-Net training 48 randomly selected images (10%) were left out for testing, the remaining 429 images were split 80/20 into 344 training and 85 validation images.

Vessel Analysis. Because ground truth masks were not available, we had a trained ophthalmologist qualitatively validate the vessel segmentation and diameter results. The results were in accordance with the experts' requirements. They found that large and medium-sized vessels are segmented reliably and their diameters are determined correctly. Small vessels were generally excluded from segmentation, as requested, with few exceptions. Only in the case of very bright image artifacts was vessel segmentation interrupted in the area of the artifact in a few cases. However, this did not compromise the ability to visually evaluate the vessel diameter and did not result in falsely detected cones. They found that large and medium-sized vessels were segmented reliably and their diameters were determined correctly. With a few exceptions, small vessels were generally segmented as required.

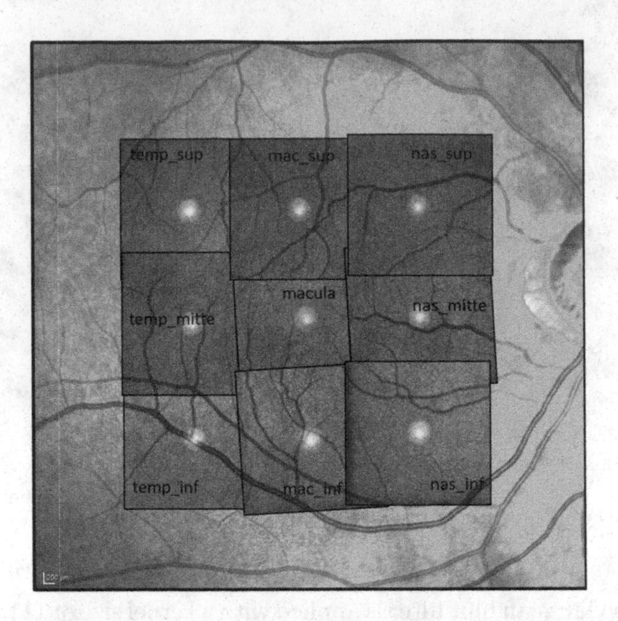

Fig. 4. Schematic illustration of scanning locations for the retina of the right eye. For the left eye these would be mirrored.

Cone Detection. The cone detection results are rated as good by the ophthalmologist, even for difficult images where it is hard to detect cones visually. As required by the physicians there were almost no false detections inside medium and large vessels. Difficulties only arise with very poor image quality. If the cones are not visually resolvable any more it also becomes virtually impossible to detect cones, both for the automatic method as well as for manual detection.

To quantitatively evaluate the performance of our cone detection method a physician manually reviewed the results of the automatic cone detection and marked falsely detected or missing cones in a total of 18 sections with a size of 380×380 px. From each, glaucoma and healthy patients, three subjects were selected at random. Care was taken to ensure that as many different image sections as possible – with and without vessels – were viewed. To validate the results, they were then checked again by a trained ophthalmologist with several years of experience. Our automatic cone detection method correctly identified cones with a mean detection rate of 0.97 and precision of 0.99 (see Table 1). Detection rate and precision are similar in both glaucoma and healthy patients.

Table 1. Evaluation of cone detection

ID	CCM	CCA	TP	FP	FN	Detection rate	Precision
Normal 0	1358	1321	1318	3	40	0.971	0.998
Normal 1	1184	1178	1174	4	10	0.992	0.997
Normal 2	1260	1231	1227	4	33	0.974	0.997
Normal 3	1361	1318	1313	5	48	0.965	0.996
Normal 4	1126	1068	1060	8	66	0.941	0.993
Normal 5	1166	1126	1120	6	46	0.961	0.995
Normal 6	1276	1229	1221	8	55	0.957	0.993
Normal 7	1215	1189	1177	12	38	0.969	0.990
Normal 8	1283	1254	1249	5	34	0.973	0.996
Glaucoma 0	636	634	629	5	7	0.989	0.992
Glaucoma 1	696	688	684	4	12	0.983	0.994
Glaucoma 2	818	798	795	3	23	0.972	0.996
Glaucoma 3	670	654	648	6	22	0.967	0.991
Glaucoma 4	778	758	746	12	32	0.959	0.984
Glaucoma 5	727	712	706	6	21	0.971	0.992
Glaucoma 6	511	504	499	5	12	0.977	0.990
Glaucoma 7	722	696	679	17	43	0.940	0.976
Glaucoma 8	736	721	712	9	24	0.967	0.988
Mean ± SD						0.968 ± 0.014	0.992 ± 0.005

CCM=Cone Count Manually, CCA=Cone Count Automatically,
TP=True Positive, FP=False Positive, FN=False Negative

4 Discussion and Conclusion

In this work we provide a comprehensive selection of methods for supporting routine questions on real clinical image data. With a mean detection rate of 0.97 and precision of 0.99 we presented a robust intensity based cone detection method (see Table 1 for details). The number of automatically counted cones is generally a little bit smaller than the cones counted by the human expert, but not to an extent that it affects the diagnostic conclusions drawn from the cone density estimation. Cone density in HMM images can be reliably determined in both images of patients with glaucoma and healthy patients. Also our proposed methods perform well on images of different quality standards, even in difficult input images, which was validated by the experts. The results are comparable to human expert performance and can be used in clinical routine.

Vessel masking ensures that cone detection results will not be corrupted by false detection inside large vessels. Vessel segmentation is also being used to automatically determine diameters of vessels from HMM images which can provide valuable insights about retinal or cardiovascular state of health.

Offering a cone density map provides additional relevant information about cone distribution in glaucoma patients and allows ophthalmologists not only to examine overall cone density in patients with or without glaucoma, but also to compare the distribution of functional and non-functional cones with a patients' field of view.

With the developed methods for estimating cone density and vessel diameter in HMM images, we have laid the foundation for further developments of helpful functionalities to support ophthalmologists in clinical routine. In the future, we will expand our work towards clinical decision support. Interesting issues in this context are detection and analysis of cone patterns over all 9 images acquired from a patient's retina during an eye examination (see Fig. 4). Correlations between vascular parameters, cone density and specific pathologies can also be further investigated using additional automated analysis methods.

References

1. Bergeles, C., et al.: Unsupervised identification of cone photoreceptors in non-confocal adaptive optics scanning light ophthalmoscope images. Biomed. Opt. Express **8**(6), 3081-3094 (2017). https://doi.org/10.1364/BOE.8.003081. http://opg.optica.org/boe/abstract.cfm?URI=boe-8-6-3081
2. Chen, Y., et al.: Automated cone cell identification on adaptive optics scanning laser ophthalmoscope images based on TV-L1 optical flow registration and k-means clustering. Appl. Sci. **11**(5) (2021). https://doi.org/10.3390/app11052259, https://www.mdpi.com/2076-3417/11/5/2259
3. Chen, Y., et al.: DeepLab and bias field correction based automatic cone photoreceptor cell identification with adaptive optics scanning laser ophthalmoscope images. Wirel. Commun. Mob. Comput. **2021**, 2034125 (2021). https://doi.org/10.1155/2021/2034125
4. Cunefare, D., Fang, L., Cooper, R.F., Dubra, A., Carroll, J., Farsiu, S.: Open source software for automatic detection of cone photoreceptors in adaptive optics ophthalmoscopy using convolutional neural networks. Sci. Rep. **7**(1), 6620 (2017). https://doi.org/10.1038/s41598-017-07103-0
5. Jonas, J.B., Schneider, U., Naumann, G.O.: Count and density of human retinal photoreceptors. Graefe's Arch. Clin. Exp. Ophthalmol. **230**(6), 505–510 (1992). https://doi.org/10.1007/BF00181769
6. Li, K.Y., Roorda, A.: Automated identification of cone photoreceptors in adaptive optics retinal images. J. Opt. Soc. Am. A Opt. Image Sci. Vis. **24**(5), 1358–1363 (2007)
7. Mariotti, L., Devaney, N.: Cone detection and blood vessel segmentation on AO retinal images (2015)
8. Mulders, T., Dhooge, P., van der Zanden, L., Hoyng, C.B., Theelen, T.: Validated filter-based photoreceptor count algorithm on retinal heidelberg high magnification module^{TM} images in healthy and pathological conditions. Appl. Sci. (Basel) **11**(12), 5347 (2021)
9. Ronneberger, O., Fischer, P., Brox, T.: U-Net: convolutional networks for biomedical image segmentation. CoRR abs/1505.04597 (2015). http://arxiv.org/abs/1505.04597
10. Xue, B., Choi, S.S., Doble, N., Werner, J.S.: Photoreceptor counting and montaging of en-face retinal images from an adaptive optics fundus camera. J. Opt. Soc. Am. A Opt. Image Sci. Vis. **24**(5), 1364–1372 (2007)

Author Index

Printed in the United States
by Baker & Taylor Publisher Services

Printed in the United States
by Baker & Taylor Publisher Services